RACE WALKING REVOLUTION

BY

JEFF SALVAGE

TIM SEAMAN

Tammy,
Best of luck,
I am sure
you'll straighten
up soon!
JS.

This book is dedicated in memory of Dr. Tom Eastler whose contributions to race walking in Maine and nationally are as countless as the individuals he touched with his generosity and kind soul. Doc Rock, you will be missed.

First Edition
ISBN: 978-1-7335757-0-6
Copyright 2019, Salvage Write Media
This book was written in conjunction with the *USA Race Walking Foundation*.
Medford, NJ

Table of Contents

Acknowledgments

Race Walking Revolution does not contain just the combined knowledge of Tim Seaman, Rachel Seaman, and Jeff Salvage, but the combined knowledge of ourselves as well as those who influenced and built our foundation of race walking knowledge. Some of our biggest influences were Ken Hendler, Gary Westerfied, Troy Engle, Frank Alongi, Jake Jacobson, Tom Eastler, Mario Fiore, Jim DiSalvo, Frank Manhardt, Bohdan Bulakowski, Enrique Peña, Mike DeWitt, Stephan Platzer, Allen James, Kevin Eastler, A.C. Jaime, Diane Graham-Henry, Paul Mascali, Ray Kuhles, Curt Clausen, Andrew Hermann, and of course Jefferson Perez. Thanks go to Luke DePron and Michael Roth for their assistance with the strength training chapter, Diane Graham-Henry for the many edits, as well as father-son team Carl / MJ Meyer for help with the cover design.

Special thanks go to my wife Jennifer who in addition to providing valuable edits, provides loving neck rubs while I camp at the computer and supports all of my efforts in race walking.

Foreword

Why is race walking becoming a trend in today's world?

It is a trend because it is physical activity with low impact that generates multiple health benefits, and it can be practiced by athletes of all ages.

Not only is race walking an Olympic sport in which the athlete pushes himself to his maximum level, race walking has also become an exclusive sport as it has no mechanical assistance other than his/her own body to move from one point to another. This allows many athletes of different countries to participate in this event, regardless of the political or economic situation of their country.

The **Race Walking Revolution** takes us on an exciting journey where experts guide us in a professional way on how to properly practice the sport. They'll provide important advice from their own experience and studies over decades that will allow us to achieve a complete holistic vision from a practical and theoretical perspective.

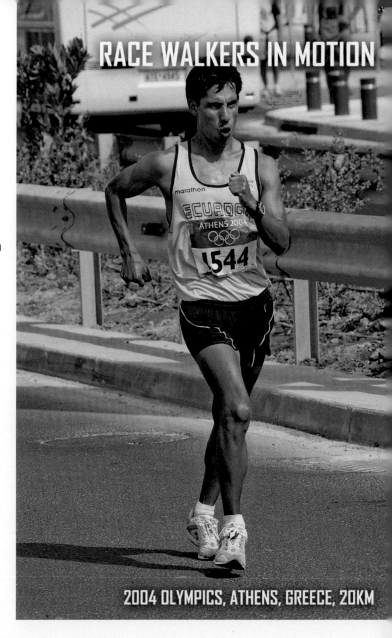

RACE WALKERS IN MOTION

2004 OLYMPICS, ATHENS, GREECE, 20KM

Enjoy this trip in the world of race walking with the guidance of passionate experts that can help you to be a better athlete and citizen and open up many opportunities in your future.

Congratulations to the authors of such wonderful work for their commitment to the development of race walking throughout the world.

Sincerely,
Jefferson Perez - Ecuador
Three Time IAAF World Champion
Olympic Gold and Silver Medalist
Former World Record Holder

RACE WALKERS IN MOTION

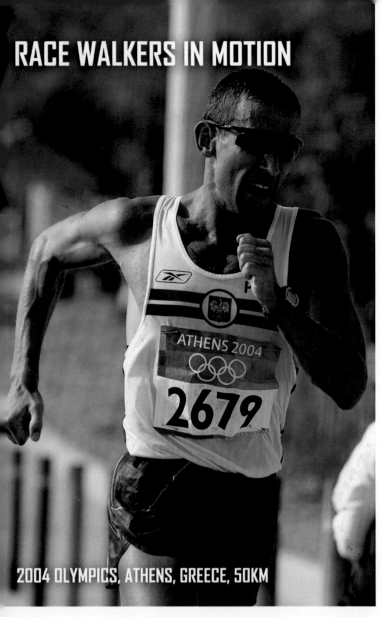

2004 OLYMPICS, ATHENS, GREECE, 50KM

As a former high performance walker and currently a track and field coach on daily basis I am involved with fitness walking for amateurs. I've founded a real tool for better walking practice in the *Race Walking Revolution*.

We all needed such revolutionary compendium of the most exercised human physical activity: race walking coaches, fitness training specialists, physiotherapists, health and sports related journalists, walking fans, or simply the people looking for their life balance. Since I've ended my high performance career in 2004 I see year after year increasing interest for better race walking understanding. Some people drop off running because of health problems caused by typical injuries of runners, others start walking because they are significantly overweight, are in the recovery stage from pregnancy or other medical recommendation. All of them need a good instruction for individual practice. Their coaches and / or therapists need the best handbook as well for walking students.

I hope that this book will really contribute to the global race walking development and better large public understanding. Congratulations for both authors Jeff Salvage and Tim Seaman for their great job and wish new international edition, the Polish one included.

Sincerely

Robert Korzeniowski, Poland
4x Olympic Gold Medalist
3x IAAF World Champion

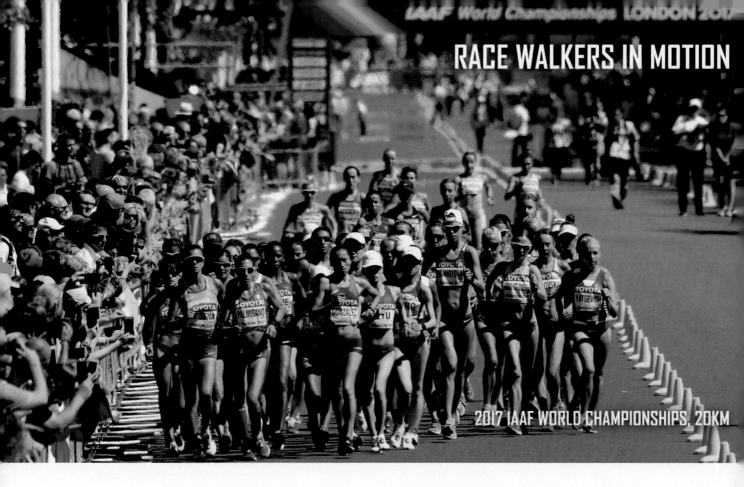

2017 IAAF WORLD CHAMPIONSHIPS, 20KM

Elite race walkers whip around the track with an unparalleled fluidity and grace. While they achieve speeds many runners would be envious of, they do so with a significantly lower incidence of injury (86% less than running). Race walking has been around in one form or another for hundreds of years. An Olympic event since 1904, amazingly, at one point in history professional walkers earned more money that professional baseball players.

Today race walkers compete from short sprints like a 1500m and mile event, to longer distances like 5km, 10km, 20km, and the longest footrace in the Olympics, the 50km.

Race walking is also great for children. It moves them off the couch, gets them active, and gives them a positive self-image. Young walkers can do it for the fun or competition with a wide set of events available.

As walkers age, their opportunities expand. Some states like New York and Maine have race walking as an event as part of the high school track and field program. NAIA colleges offer scholarships with plenty of opportunities to compete. If there are no scholastic programs near you, there are countless walking clubs to provide camaraderie and advice.

While race walking can be started early, it is not limited to the young. Many masters athletes compete in their age group at events across the country or internationally. Unlike non-weight bearing sports like swimming, the low impact nature of race walking helps prevent osteoporosis by strengthening the bones without the high risk of injuries from more aggressive exercises.

For my father, exercise was a spectator sport and not something to participate in. As he aged, his life-long lack of activity severely limited his quality of life.

When you think of someone old, what comes to mind? Someone who is frail and has a lack of range of motion in their gait. Race walkers are the antithesis of this. They drive their legs, arms, and hips threw a full-range of motion unseen in most forms of exercise. They power forward with a combination of locomotion that utilizes all the body's muscles.

So, are you ready to join the *Race Walking Revolution*? If so, please read on, but please consult a doctor before starting any exercise program.

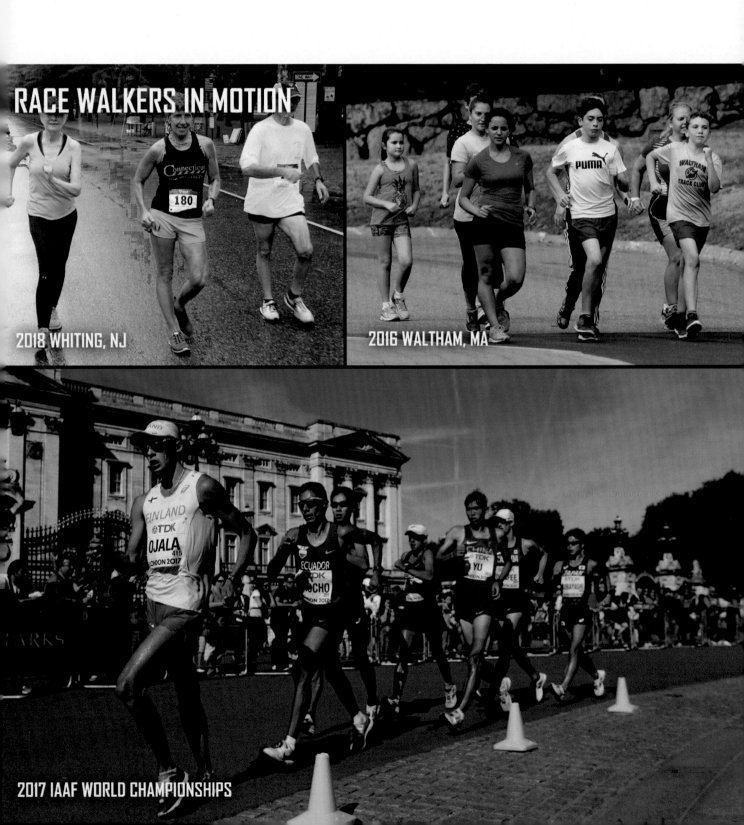

RACE WALKERS IN MOTION

2018 WHITING, NJ

2016 WALTHAM, MA

2017 IAAF WORLD CHAMPIONSHIPS

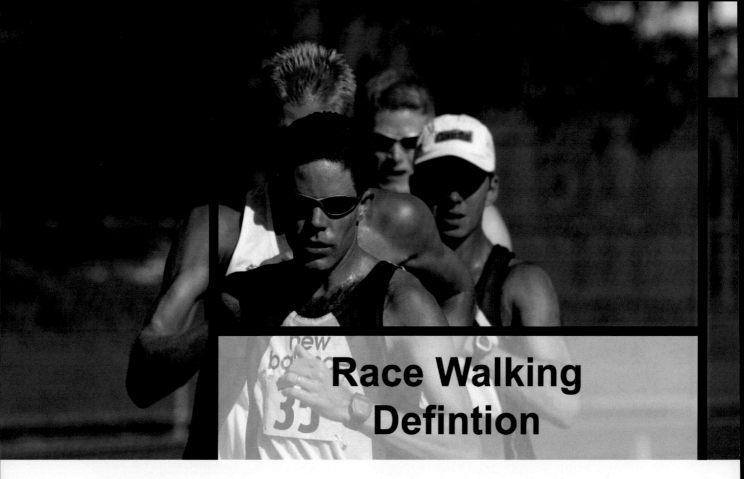

Race Walking Defintion

When in high school, I was introduced to the sport of race walking after a series of running injuries derailed my high school running efforts. I took an instant love to the exhilaration and challenges provided by race walking. The intensity from driving my arms, swinging my hips, and the fast turnover of my legs got my heart going both literally and figuratively. My injuries greatly reduced, and I excelled competitively in ways I never imagined. Now, well into middle age, my competitive juices are gone, but I race walk regularly to stay fit and healthy.

Tim also started race walking in high school to help his team win points at dual meets. Always the team player, Tim did what the coach asked. Two years later, Tim received a scholarship to the University of Wisconsin - Parkside and he won his first U.S. Junior Championship. He went on to having one of the most successful competitive race walking careers in the USA that included berths on two Olympic teams and 47 national titles. He has since retired from competitive walking, but is highly active coaching athletes including 7 that competed in the Olympics.

Rachel Seaman also got an early start. At 16, she was caught making fun of her older sister who was race walking on the Canadian National Junior team and challenged to try it herself. She has since qualified for one Olympic team and is currently training for her second.

Between the three of us, the *Race Walk Revolution* book encompassed a combined 80+ years of experience in race walking. Together, we provide an unparalleled approach to learning race walking regardless of whether you are a young walker learning to participate, a masters athlete looking to compete in your age group, an inspiring Olympian, or a recreational walker of any age that wants to amplify your walking workout in a safe and efficient manner.

Understanding race walking starts with comprehending the definition agreed upon by both the U.S. and international track and field communities. It is:

- Race walking is a progression of steps so taken that the walker makes contact with the ground so that no visible (to the human eye) loss of contact occurs.
- The advancing leg must be straightened (i.e., not bent at the knee) from the moment of first contact with the ground until in the vertical upright position.

Whether you wish to compete or just walk for fitness, following the official definition of race walking is the best form of athletic walking. Following the definition leads to a smooth and efficient stride, with lower incidences of injuries, and a lot of time saved while working out.

While the definition of race walking may seem straightforward, it is open to a lot of interpretation. Let's start by looking at the first part of the definition. In concept it is simple. If you always have one foot on the ground, you are legal. Beginning race walkers usually always have a foot on the ground.

Some walkers, especially those who are less fit or overweight, have a prolonged portion of the stride where both feet are on the ground simultaneously (Figure 2-1). This makes it easy for a judge to observe there is no loss of contact. Notice how the rear foot hasn't rolled up onto the big toe yet. While this doesn't violate the definition of race walking, it is less efficient and can increase your chance of injuries. In contrast, the walker on the right has a momentary double-support phase (Figure 2-2). This is often considered "classic" race walking form.

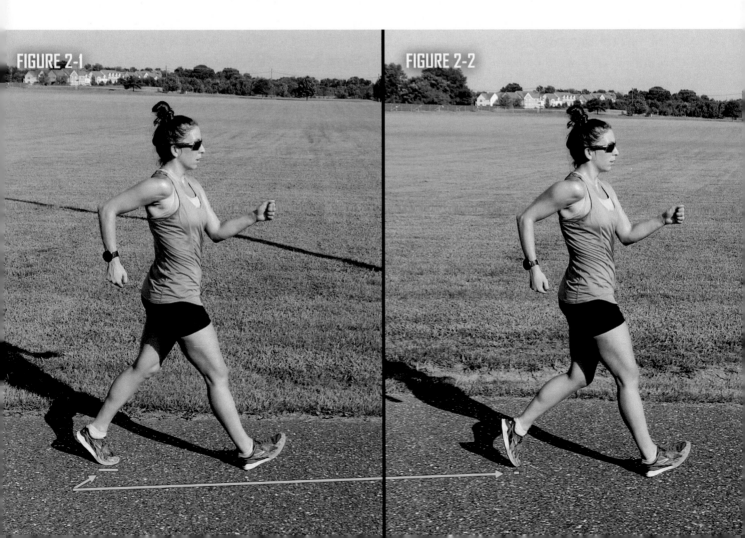

FIGURE 2-1   FIGURE 2-2

While the definition allows for a slight flight phase, there are many interpretations as to how far off the ground a race walker can be while still not having a visible, to the human eye, loss of contact.

Observe two images of Olympian Miranda Melville taken in practice and one from an international competition side by side. Each has a flight phase.

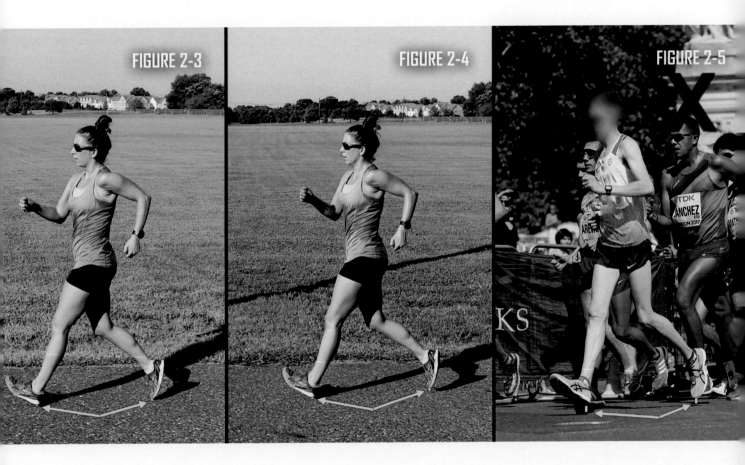

The leftmost walker (Figure 2-3) is barely off the ground and we consider that she is walking with perfectly legal form.

The middle walker (Figure 2-4) has a slightly larger flight phase, but not enough to be discerned by the human eye.

In our opinion the walker on the right (Figure 2-5) is flagrantly off the ground, by enough to be visible to the human eye. Therefore, the rightmost walker is in violation of the definition of race walking and was disqualified from the race.

The second part of the definition requires the leg to be fully extended from the moment the foot first makes contact with the ground (Figure 2-6), until the supporting leg is in the vertical upright position (Figure 2-7). The idea is simple, however, in practice it takes a degree of dexterity, muscle strength and flexibility.

While the rules only state you must have your leg straightened until vertical, there are advantages to maintaining a straightened leg longer (Figure 2-8).

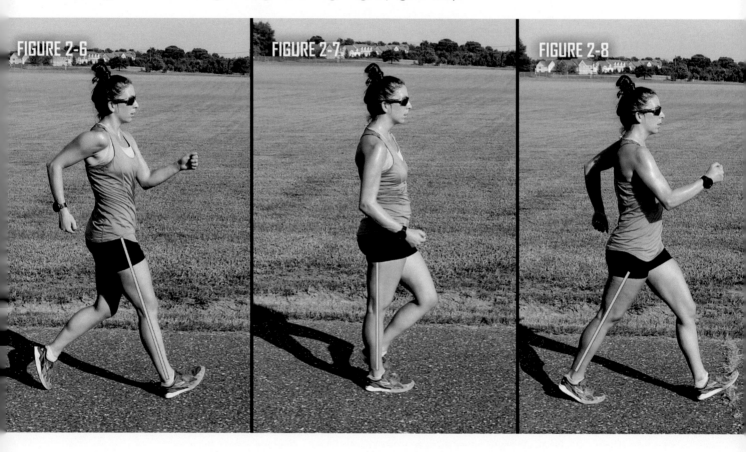

FIGURE 2-6   FIGURE 2-7   FIGURE 2-8

Amazingly, if you want to be a legal race walker, that's all you have to do.

However, there are many subtle aspects of a race walker's stride that are worth learning to maximize your efficiency and speed. Therefore, we will continue by dissecting every aspect of race walking technique.

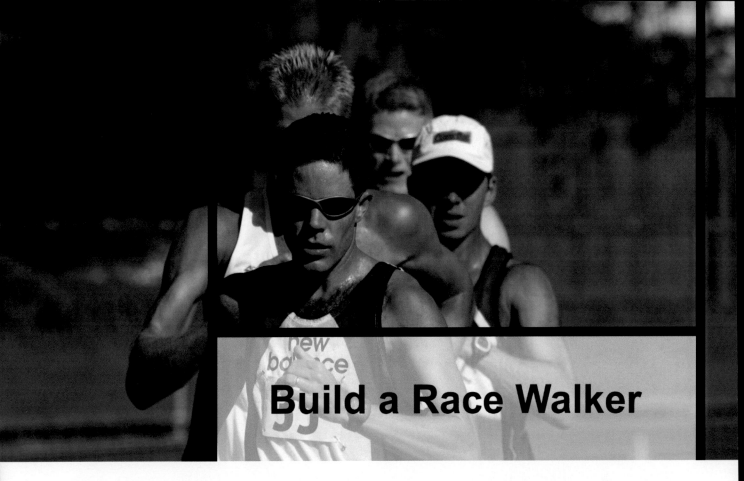

Build a Race Walker

When we instruct our clinics, we like to start our hands-on session of teaching race walking with **Build a Race Walker**. First, we demonstrate what good race walking is and do so with an explanation from the top of the body down. A walker's head should be looking straight ahead (Figure 3-1), not down or tilted to the side. The shoulders should be relaxed, the arms held at roughly 90 degrees with the hands swinging from just behind the hip to the center of the sternum (Figure 3-2). While the arms swing back and forth, it's important for the angle of the upper and lower arm to remain constant and not open on the back swing or close on the swing forward.

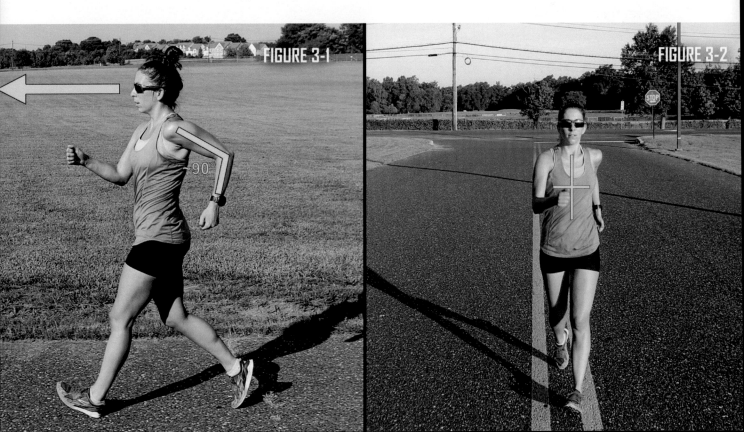

FIGURE 3-1

FIGURE 3-2

Most newcomers to race walking have no issue keeping one foot on the ground at all times, but they do struggle with swinging the legs through properly and mastering straightening of the knee. Therefore, given these challenges and that the definition of race walking only stipulates conditions on the legs and feet, **Build a Race Walker** focuses on the lower body in three phases.

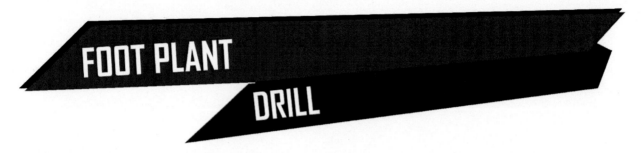

FOOT PLANT DRILL

The first 10% of the stride is most important. It's what helps differentiate a race walker from a speed or health walker. It focuses on heel strike with the toe pointed up. We call it the **Foot Plant** drill and you must master it before progressing forward.

STEPS

1. Start by standing with your weight on your rear foot (Figure 3-3).
2. Swing your other leg forward (Figure 3-4) from the knee until it fully extends.
3. As you do, land with your foot slightly in front of the body, with your toes up and the knee straightened (Figure 3-5).
4. Transfer all your weight to that leg (Figure 3-6).
5. While virtually standing in place, rock back and forth from one foot to the other emphasizing the heel strike.
6. Note that the knee does bend when you rock back.
7. Repeat this exercise for both legs.

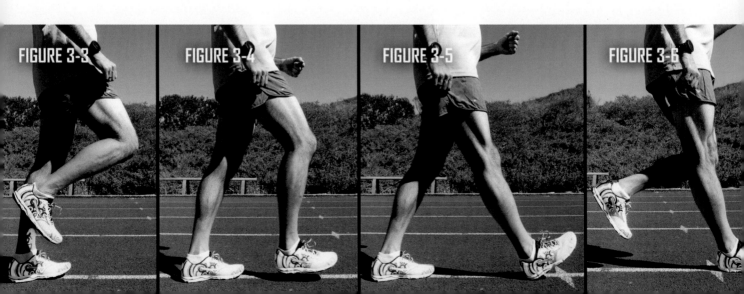

FIGURE 3-3   FIGURE 3-4   FIGURE 3-5   FIGURE 3-6

PUSH OFF DRILL

Next, we segue to the last 10% of the stride known as **_Push Off_**. This is a slow walking exercise.

STEPS

1. Start with your forward foot's toes on the ground with forward leg's knee straightened, and its heel planted on the ground; In addition, the rear leg is also straightened (Figure 3-7).
2. Reach forward with the forward leg, land on your heel, with your toes pointed; simultaneously, push off the rear foot, lifting the heel off the ground (Figure 3-8).
3. Unlike a race walking stride, place your rear foot back on the ground about 12 inches from where it toed off.
4. Repeat this exercise with both legs.

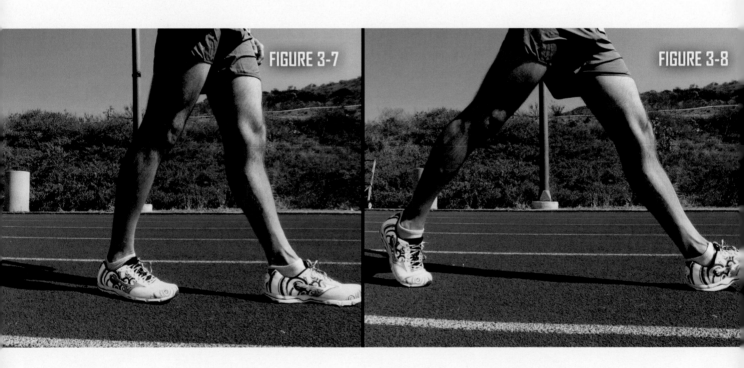

FIGURE 3-7

FIGURE 3-8

LEG SWING DRILL

What's left is what happens in the middle.

STEPS

1. Once you push off the rear foot (Figure 3-9), you must rapidly swing the leg forward into the attack position.
2. Practice swinging the leg forward quickly (Figure 3-10), extending the knee fully, as fast as possible (Figure 3-11).
3. As you swing the leg forward, focus on keeping the foot very low to the ground.
4. Repeat this exercise with both legs.

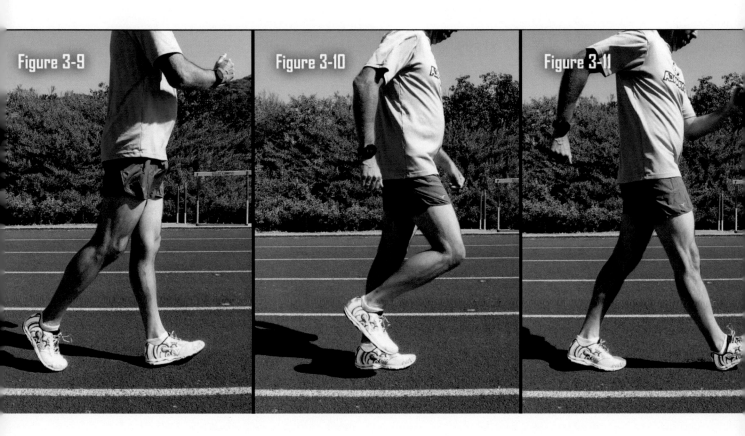

Figure 3-9　　　Figure 3-10　　　Figure 3-11

SIMPLE ARMS DRILL

Now that the lower body is set, let's do a quick lesson on arms.

STEPS

1. Stand in place and swing your arms through the proper race walking motion with your hands swinging from your sternum all the way back behind your hips (Figure 3-11).
2. When they do, focus on keeping the angle between the upper and lower arm to approximately 90 degrees and locked in place (Figure 3-12).
3. Also, focus on relaxing the shoulders.

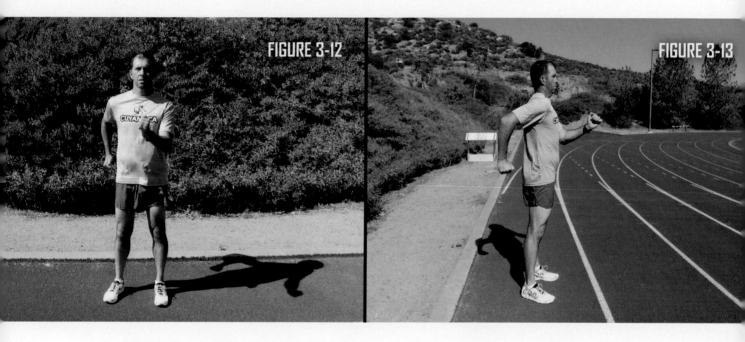

FIGURE 3-12

FIGURE 3-13

With these basic tutorials in place you are now ready to put them all together and race walk.

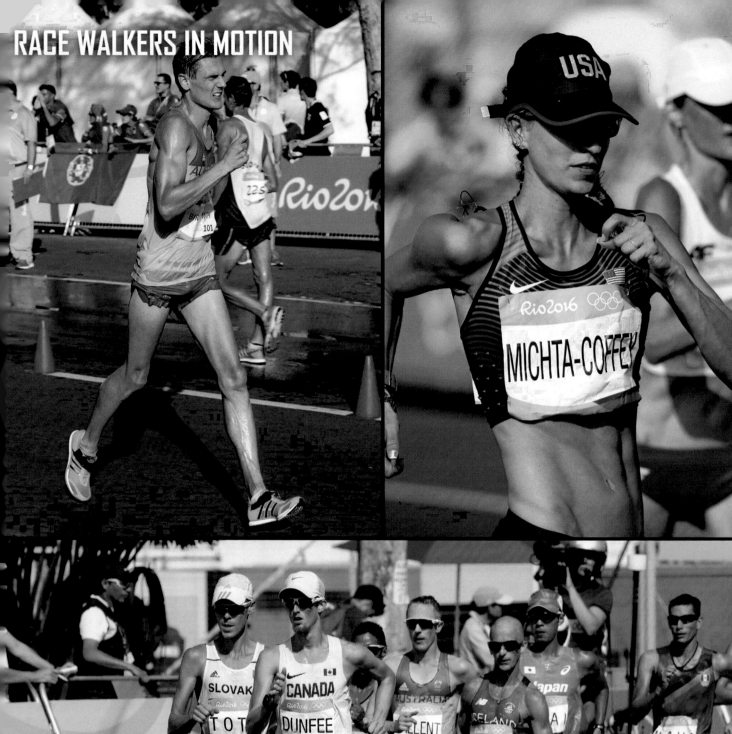

RACE WALKERS IN MOTION

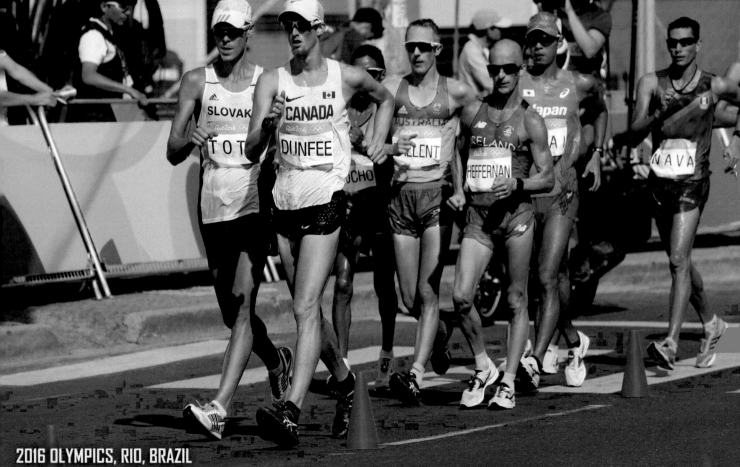

2016 OLYMPICS, RIO, BRAZIL

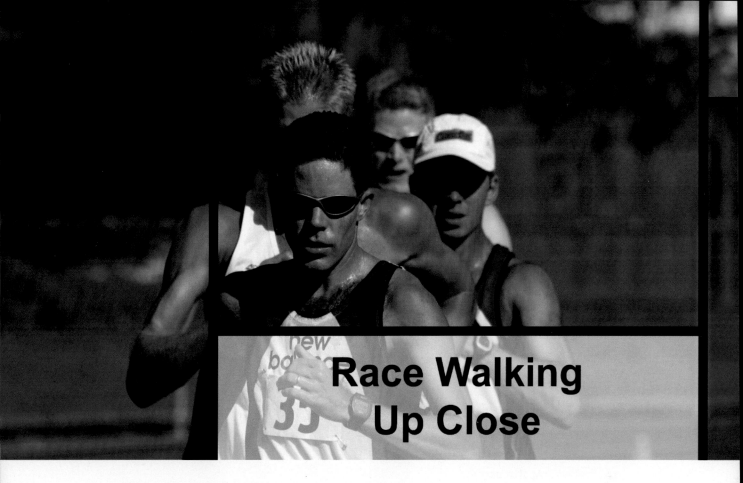

Race Walking Up Close

Let's look at race walking in more detail. While the definition of race walking is fairly concise, the nuances and complexities of efficient race walking technique are far from simple. Watching elite walkers blaze by leaves you awestruck. It also leaves you with an image of textbook form that is fluid, powerful, and graceful. While many positive adjectives can replace those stated, they don't describe why race walkers look so good. The key to good form is a combination of strength and range of motion.

Before we dive in, a brief a note about our explanation. When we state average statistics, we are not simply making up numbers. We studied high frame rate video and sequenced still photographs of many of the best race walkers in the world. Our numbers are an average of those findings. If you are interested in the details of the study, please read **Looking at the Best, A Detailed Analysis of Elite Race Walking Technique**.

STEP RATIO

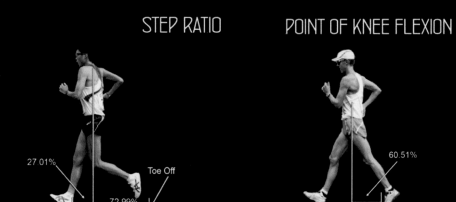

27.01%

Toe Off

72.99%

POINT OF KNEE FLEXION

60.51%

AVERAGE LOSS OF CONTACT

2.85 cm (1.12 Inches) Off the Ground

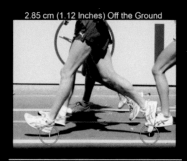

Posture

Let's start our discussion with posture. Notice how a race walker's torso is in a vertical position (Figures 4-2 through 4-7). Historically, this wasn't always the case with race walkers coached to lean from the ankles. This led to a very sore lower back as well as restricted hip rotation. By walking tall, walkers technique is more graceful and efficient. Their posture is one factor in why they can achieve the ideal of having a longer stride behind the body than in front of the body.

Overall Stride

Let's observe a complete stride. We can see the right foot striking the ground at the heel while the leg simultaneously straightens (Figure 4-2), the leg stays straightened as the body passes directly over the leg (Figure 4-4) and beyond (Figure 4-6). Finally, the leg bends (Figure 4-7) as the ball of the right foot begins to lift from the ground. The leg then swings forward until it straightens in front of the body as the heel contacts the ground. Achieving this smooth, synchronized action is the key to success.

Let's dissect the stride further by observing what happens as the leg completes its swing forward. As it straightens the toes are pointed up (between 20 to 30 degrees from the ground as measured along the sole of the shoe) and the heel strikes the ground (Figure 4-1).

FIGURE 4

~20-30°

Then the body moves forward over the right leg. This is where walkers tend to violate the definition of race walking. The leg must remain straightened until it is in the vertical position.

Once the leg is beyond the vertical position, it may bend.

However, when it comes time to lift your heel off the ground, if your leg is still straightened, you get an extra thrust forward by pushing off your rear foot. With proper flexibility and strength your leg stays straightened longer, and you obtain this advantageous thrust. Ideally, the leg remains straightened until the ball of your rear foot is about to lift off the ground.

Then roll up onto the toe of your rear foot. Notice that as the rear (right) foot leaves the ground, the front (left) leg is already in position (Figure 4-7).

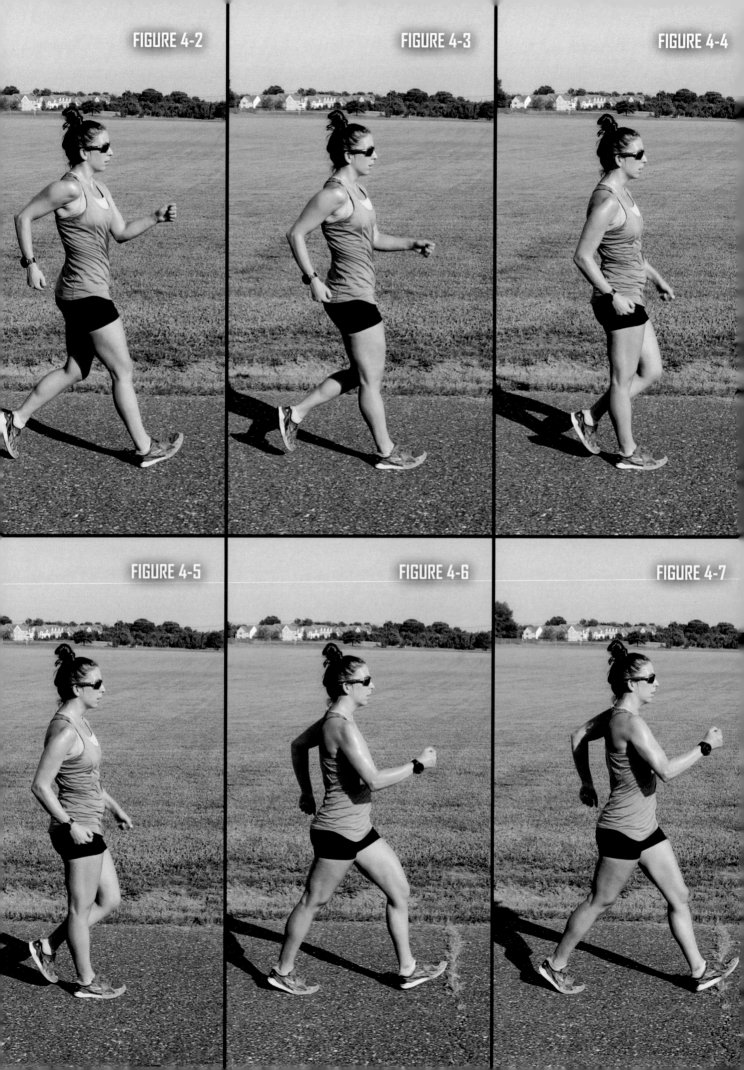

FIGURE 4-2

FIGURE 4-3

FIGURE 4-4

FIGURE 4-5

FIGURE 4-6

FIGURE 4-7

Let's also note the position of the rest of the body. The right arm swings backward coming up to an angle of 20-30 degrees (Figure 4-8). While for decades we've stated you should hold your arms at 90 degrees, most elite walkers hold there are angle at slightly less than 90 degree.

The key is for your hand to swing to just behind the hip (Figure 4-9). If you are holding your arm at 85 degrees and it's not swinging back far enough, try opening your arm angle to 90 or 95 degrees. In contrast, if your hand is not coming far enough back, then open the arm angle until you achieve proper hand position. The variation can be for many reasons including a difference in the ratio between your upper and lower arm.

Finally note the ratio of the stride in front and behind the body. It should be roughly 40/60 (Figure 4-10). Note, when elite walkers gain a flight phase it can be closer to 30/70. The legs do not create a symmetrical triangle. This is achieved through proper hip action, which is explained shortly. How you measure it matters. In this case we are measuring the front of the stride from the point of heel contact to the center of the torso and the rear portion from the center of the torso to the point of toe off.

Having less of your stride in front of the body allows a walker to optimize their stride by having more of the stride in the propulsive phase. In contrast, when the foot is on the ground and too far in front of the body it acts as a brake, slowing the walker's progress as well as adding stress that can lead to injuries.

Next, we observe the right leg as it swings forward (Figure 4-11 through 4-16). The goal is for the foot to swing forward as low to the ground as possible. This averts loss of contact problems that might occur if you drive your foot too high coming through your stride. If your foot is too high, you might have a propensity to drive the leg up instead of forward, thus making you at risk of visible loss of contact and getting disqualified. Watch the progression as the rear foot leaves the ground until just after the same foot strikes the ground in front of the body.

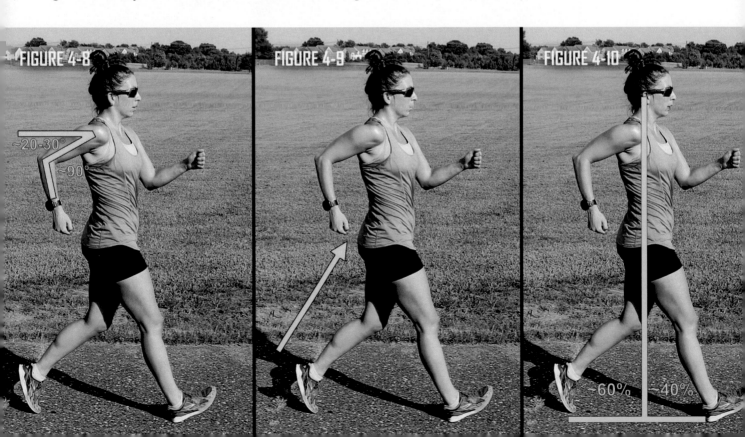

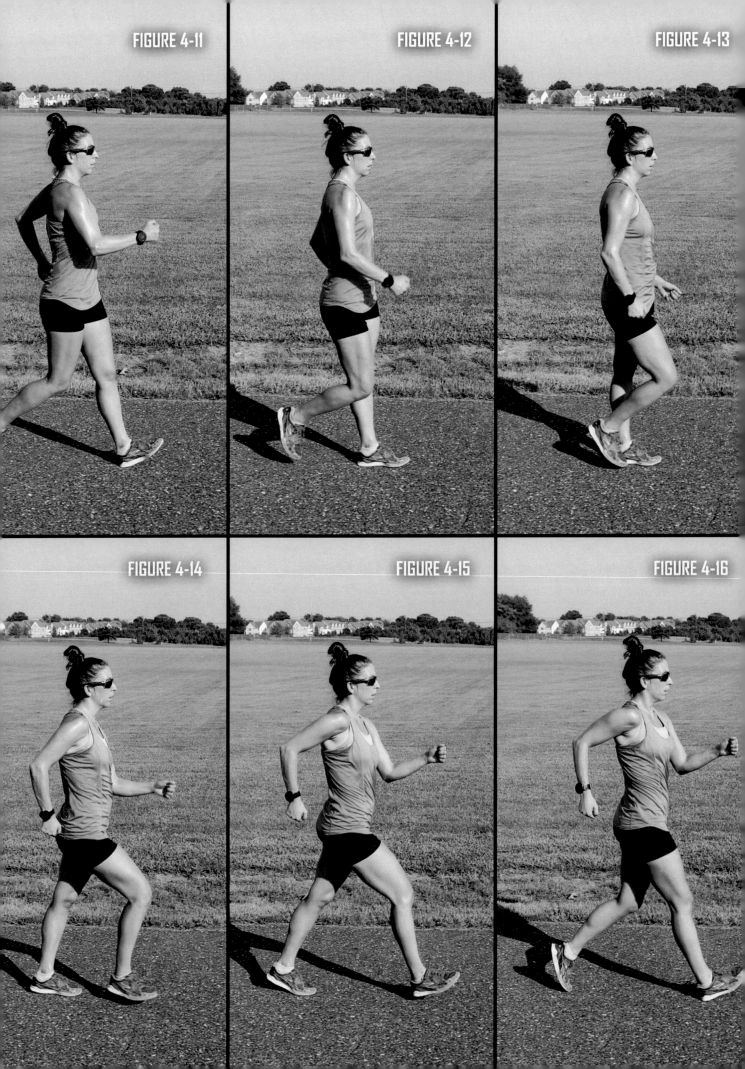

FIGURE 4-11

FIGURE 4-12

FIGURE 4-13

FIGURE 4-14

FIGURE 4-15

FIGURE 4-16

Let's look at that portion of the stride again. When the rear foot leaves the ground (4-17), it swings forward with the leg flexed at the knee (4-18, 4-19). Note the constant angle between the upper and lower leg during this phase.

When a race walker begins straightening the leg (Figure 4-14 through 4-16) as it moves forward, the quadriceps are used to extend it. When the foot makes contact with the ground, the leg must be straightened and no longer flexed at the knee.

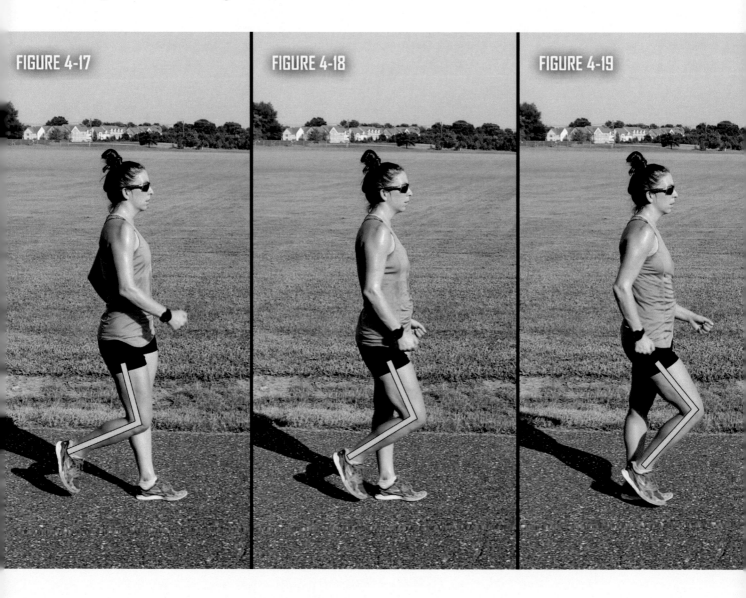

FIGURE 4-17   FIGURE 4-18   FIGURE 4-19

Let's also look closely how the foot moves forward during the swing phase (Figure 4-20). The foot hugs just above the ground. This is ideal for efficiency and the appearance of legality.

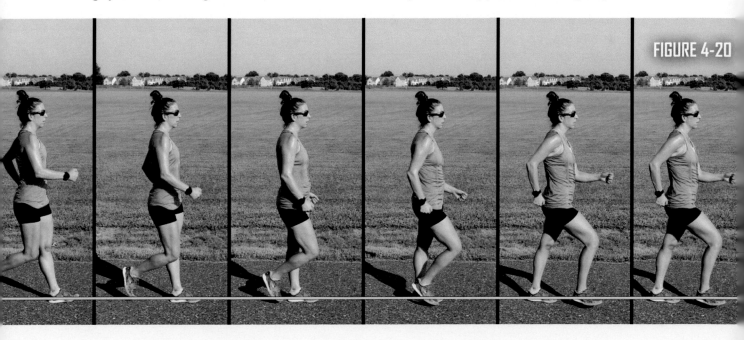

FIGURE 4-20

Let's look at a race walker from an aerial view (Figure 4-21). Notice how his footfalls land in a straight line. A pedestrian walker in contrast has footfalls on either side of a straight line (Figure 4-22). If you told a pedestrian walker to speed up, his foot falls would naturally land closer to a center line. This is because of the added engagement of the hips. The more a walker's hips engage the more the walker's feet land in a straight line.

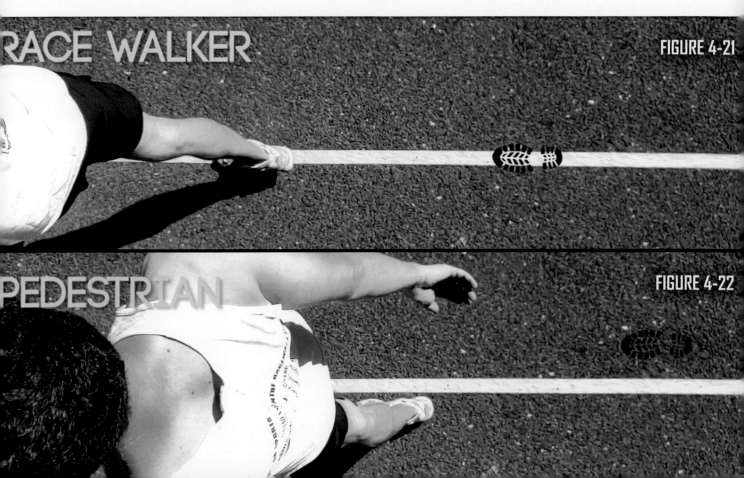

RACE WALKER

FIGURE 4-21

PEDESTRIAN

FIGURE 4-22

If we look at a walker from the front (Figure 4-23 through 4-25), we also notice that the foot does not come down flat. Instead the foot lands on the outer corner of the heel and progresses forward slowly with a natural roll to the outside of the foot. This is not forced and something to notice more than actively pursue.

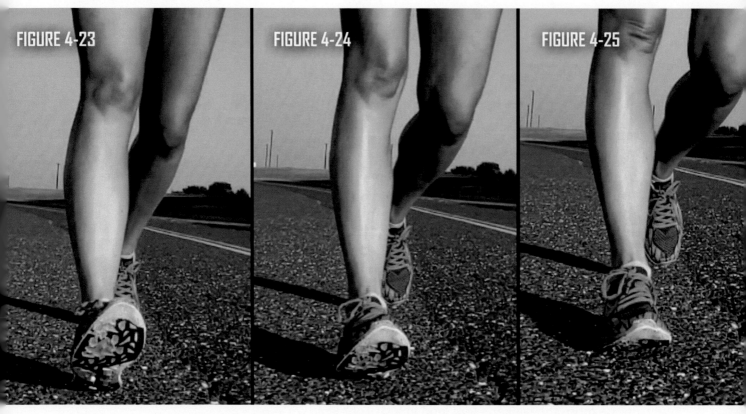

FIGURE 4-23 FIGURE 4-24 FIGURE 4-25

Finally, we can look at the walker from the back and see how the foot progresses forward (Figures 4-26 through 4-28). We can see the foot rolling forward, up on its big toe. Once the walker toes off the ground, the foot progresses forward as low to the ground as possible. The foot moves forward, while not swaying farther out than necessary.

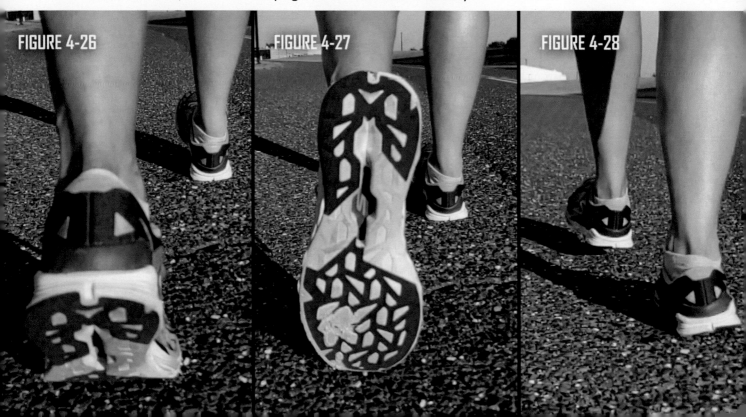

FIGURE 4-26 FIGURE 4-27 FIGURE 4-28

Hips

Elite race walkers generate their primary source of forward locomotion from rotating the hips. Repeatedly pivoting the hips forward causes them to act as the body's motor, propelling it forward one step at a time. Actively swinging the hip forward lengthens the stride from the top of the legs, while increasing stride length behind the body.

In a flexible race walker, the gain can be as much as three inches per stride. If you add as little as 1 inch to a typical 1-meter race walking stride, the net gain is approximately 10 meters per lap on a track. In a 20km race, that totals to over 500 meters gained. At an elite level, the savings is close to two minutes. In the last three Olympic Games it made the difference between a gold medal and finishing well off the podium.

An efficient race walker has more of their stride behind their body than the front. This is directly due to hip rotation. Good forward hip rotation is a key solid race walking technique.

The value of pursuing increased stride length was illustrated when Tim Seaman trained with Jefferson Perez, the 1996 Olympic champion and 2008 Olympic silver medalist. They measured their stride lengths and found that, while Jefferson is shorter than Tim, Jefferson's stride length was 1.25 meters and Tim's was 1.11 meters. That corresponds to Tim having to take 18,000 steps in a 20km race and Jefferson having to take only 16,000.

Observe the Figure 4-29 and 4-30. Both show the stride of the same race walker. The difference is the walker in Figure 4-30 is properly utilizing his hips, while the walker in Figure 4-29 is underutilizing them. Looking at the two photos, the difference is subtle. However, when comparing the strides side by side (Figure 4-31) the difference in stride length when utilizing proper hip rotation is obvious.

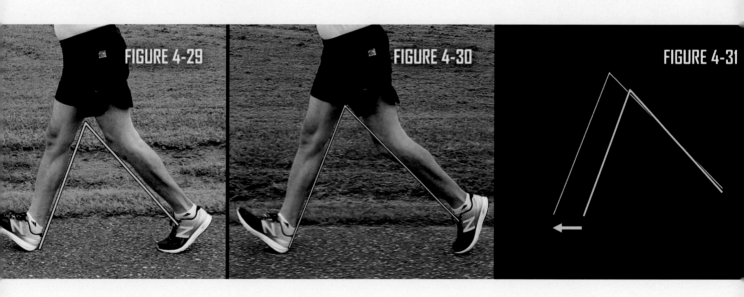

FIGURE 4-29   FIGURE 4-30   FIGURE 4-31

Some coaches tout that increasing hip rotation decreases a race walker's cadence. This is an inaccurate evaluation of biomechanics. The hip rotates forward at the same time as the leg swings forward. The leg does not swing forward before the hip rotates. Since the two motions occur simultaneously, any reduction in cadence is minimal and greatly outweighed by the increase in stride length.

The exact motion of the hips during race walking is a bit complicated. The hip moves in three dimensions; its primary movement is forward, but it also must move slightly in and out as well as up and down. To further understand proper technique, observe the hip motion from varying perspectives.

A small circular sticker on the outside of the center of the hip is a great way to observe how the hip moves as the walker progresses through the stride. We start with the center point of the right hip as a race walker plants his heel on the ground (Figure 4-32).

As the body moves forward over a straightened leg, the center point of the hip rises until the straightened leg passes directly beneath the body (Figure 4-33).

From the moment the leg passes under the body until the right foot's toe pushes off the ground, the center point of the hip moves downwards (Figure 4-34).

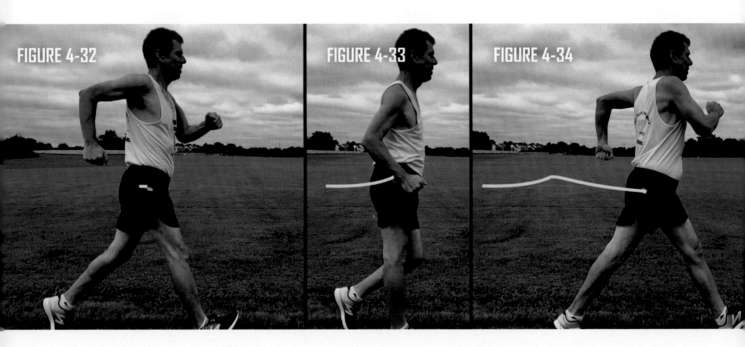

FIGURE 4-32   FIGURE 4-33   FIGURE 4-34

As the rear foot starts to swing forward, the leg must be bent (Figure 4-35).

This bent leg swings forward as the hip continues to lower slightly (Figure 4-36). This is known as "hip drop" and, while necessary, is a minimal action.

After the knee of the swing leg passes under the body (Figure 4-37), the center point of the hip rises to the neutral position (Figure 4-38).

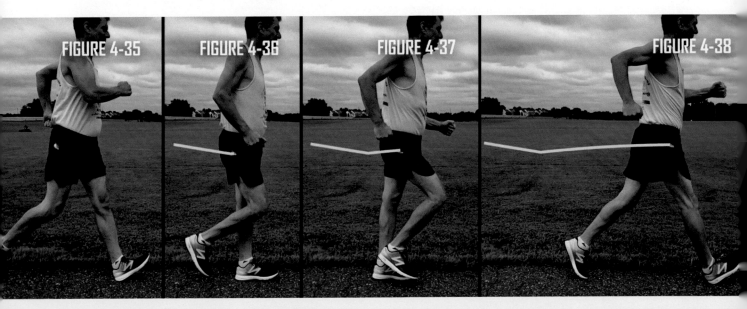

FIGURE 4-35   FIGURE 4-36   FIGURE 4-37   FIGURE 4-38

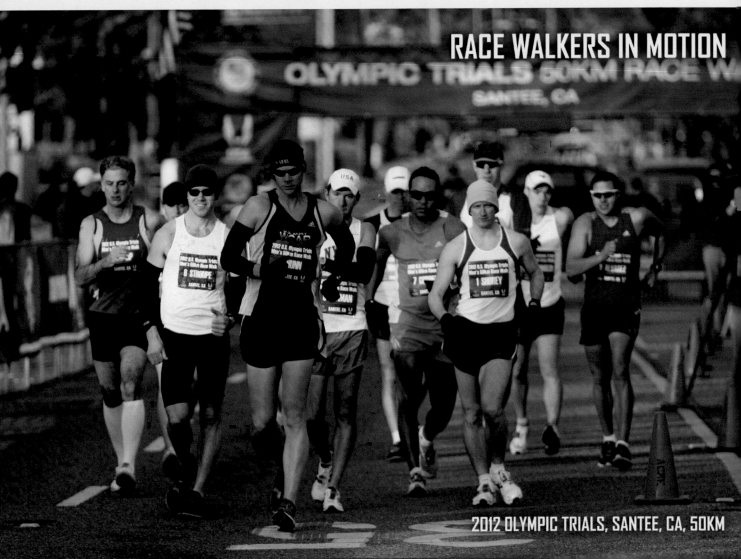

RACE WALKERS IN MOTION
OLYMPIC TRIALS 50KM RACE W
SANTEE, CA

2012 OLYMPIC TRIALS, SANTEE, CA, 50KM

To further understand the motion of the hips, let's observe the center point of the left hip of a race walker's stride as viewed from the side while the race walker is on a treadmill.

The walker's heel strikes the ground as the center point of the hip is in the neutral position (Figure 4-39).

As the treadmill carries the straightened leg backward, the center point of the hip rises (Figure 4-40). In our illustration, the center point moves clockwise.

From the moment the straightened leg passes under the body until the right foot's toe pushes off the treadmill, the center point of the hip moves down (Figure 4-41). As the rear foot begins to move forward, the leg must be bent. While it does, the hip continues to lower. This is known as "hip drop."

After the knee of the swing leg passes under the body, the center point of the hip rises to its starting position for heel strike (Figure 4-42).

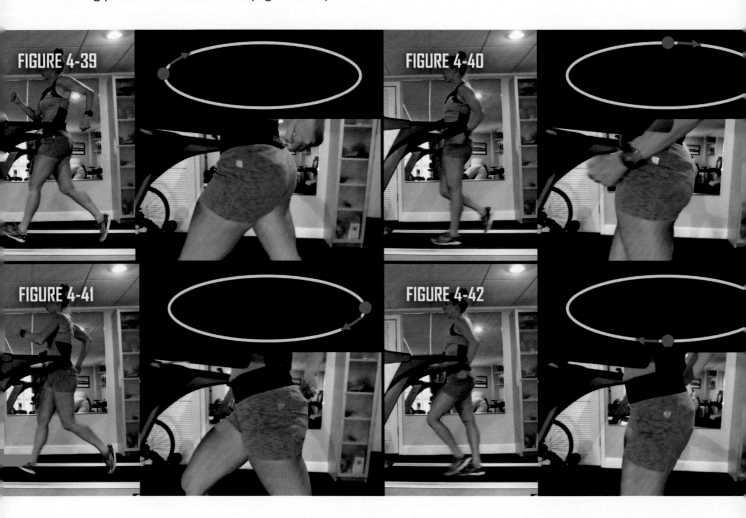

FIGURE 4-39

FIGURE 4-40

FIGURE 4-41

FIGURE 4-42

Finally, to show how the hip arcs out slightly at parts of the stride, observe a walker from a top view. Note that the outward sway is minimal and not a forced action. Instead, the hips sway in or out due to the forces subjected to it by the legs, arms, and torso.

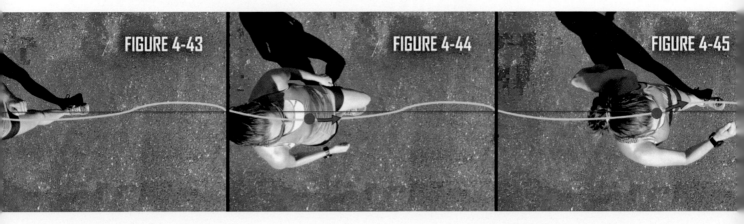

FIGURE 4-43   FIGURE 4-44   FIGURE 4-45

As the walker's left foot is about to leave the ground with the left hip behind the body, the left hip begins moving forward (Figure 4-43). As it does, it arcs out slightly (Figure 4-44).

Once the knee swings under the body, the hip continues forward while arcing inward back to the starting position (Figure 4-45).

The process is repeated when the right leg swings forward and the right hip arches outward and then backward to the neutral position.

Even after a technical explanation many beginning walkers still do not know what it should feel like to race walk with proper hip motion. When Tim and I teach race walking clinics we resort to analogies to try to get walkers to engage their hips.

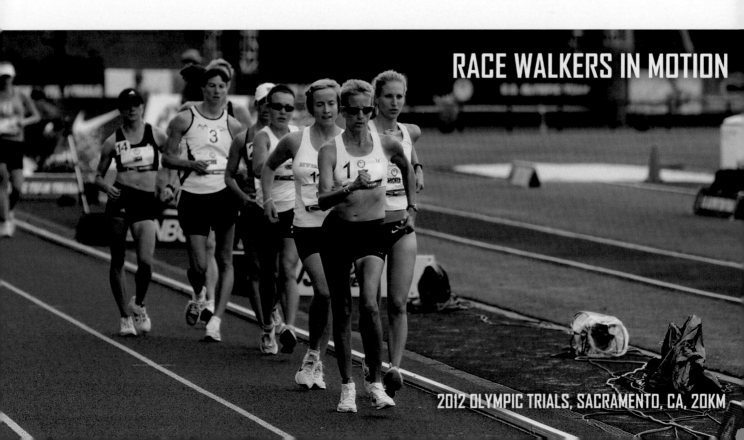

RACE WALKERS IN MOTION

2012 OLYMPIC TRIALS, SACRAMENTO, CA, 20KM

VAMPIRE IN A COFFIN
DRILL

Even though you may not feel like you are using your hips when you race walk, you are to a minimal extent. Our goal is to get you to feel what rotating your hips forward feels like.

Try this exercise, preferably at the base of a hill.

BODY POSITION

Stand like you would to start race walking.

STEPS

1. Place your hands over your chest as a vampire would in a coffin.
2. Start race walking up the hill (Figure 4-46 & Figure 4-47).
3. Make sure you use proper technique in your lower body and straighten your leg appropriately.
4. Race walk up the hill for 50 feet or so.
5. Now, accelerate your race walk; You should feel a slight tugging in your hip as it naturally begins to rotate forward.
6. Go with the feeling.
7. Exaggerate the feeling while continuing to hold your arms against your chest and straighten your leg properly.
8. After about 50 feet of accelerating, lower your arms into proper race walking position and race walk using your new exaggerated hip motion. Ideally, if you can time the lowering of your arms to reaching the top of the hill and can walk on level ground you will have the best results.

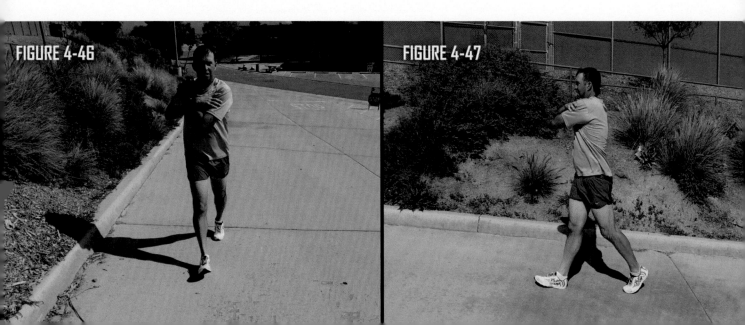

FIGURE 4-46   FIGURE 4-47

GUNSLINGER DRILL

The first analogy is to think of yourself as a gun slinger in the old west with a pistol on each hip (Figure 4-48). Imagine you want to walk thru a set of saloon doors that have a gap in the middle. However, you are not going to push the doors open with your hand. Instead, keeping your torso as still as possible, swing your right hip forward so the gun pops the door forward. Then repeat it with the left hip. Use the same hip motion when you race walk and lead your leg forward from the hip.

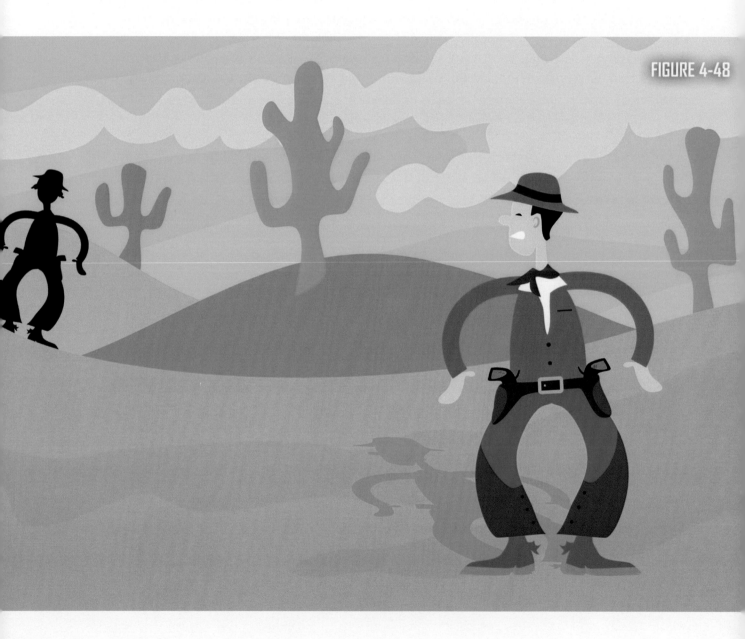

FIGURE 4-48

Arms

An elite race walker synchronizes arm and hip motion to maximize efficiency and speed. While the exact range of motion for the arm varies slightly with speed and effort, each arm travels from a couple of inches behind the hip to just above the chest line (Figure 4-49).

Notice how when the arm swings forward, the wrist is positioned above the ankle (Figure 4-50). The primary power for arm movement is derived from the backward swing of your arm. It is not a wild pumping action and does not require much effort to thrust the arm forward.

The shoulders need to be relaxed, allowing the shoulders to act as a fulcrum with the arms swinging like a pendulum.

With the proper angle, when you drive back, the arm swings to the proper position a few inches behind your hip. With a relaxed shoulder, your arm recoils forward to the correct location.

The cycle repeats with another drive of the arm backward. You'll be surprised how little effort is required to move your arm quickly. But note, your arms move only as fast as your hips and legs; it's all about synchronizing. Observe closely and you can also see how the shoulders and torso move slightly forward as the opposite hip rotates forward.

As the walker's left foot contacts the ground her right shoulder moves slightly in front of her left. You can also notice the forward presence of the right side of her torso as it counters the left hip's forward progression (Figure 4-50).

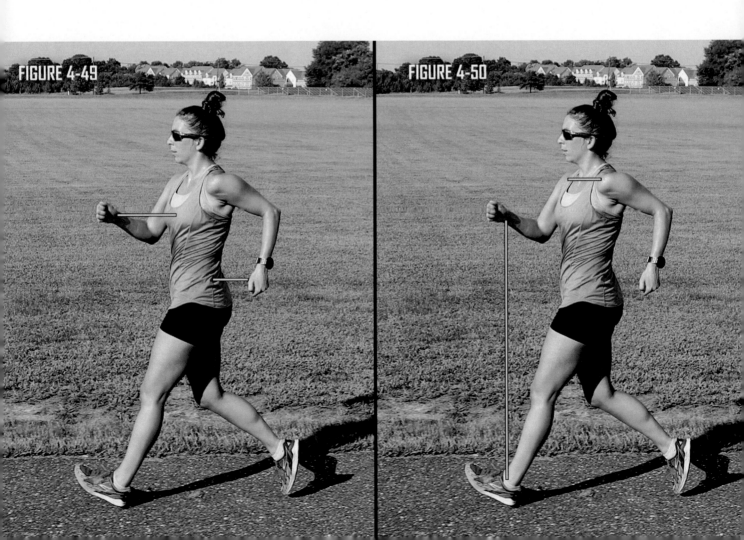

FIGURE 4-49   FIGURE 4-50

Proper arm swing must also consider how the arm crosses in front of the body. Observe how the arm swings forward as if shaking someone's hand (Figures 4-51 & 4-52). One key to good arms is to relax the shoulders. While the shoulders do move slightly forward and back, counteracting the forward hip rotation, they should remain relatively still. Observe the height of your shoulders and check whether they are relaxed. Simply place one hand on your shoulder and lower it as far down as it can go. When your shoulder is all the way down, it is relaxed.

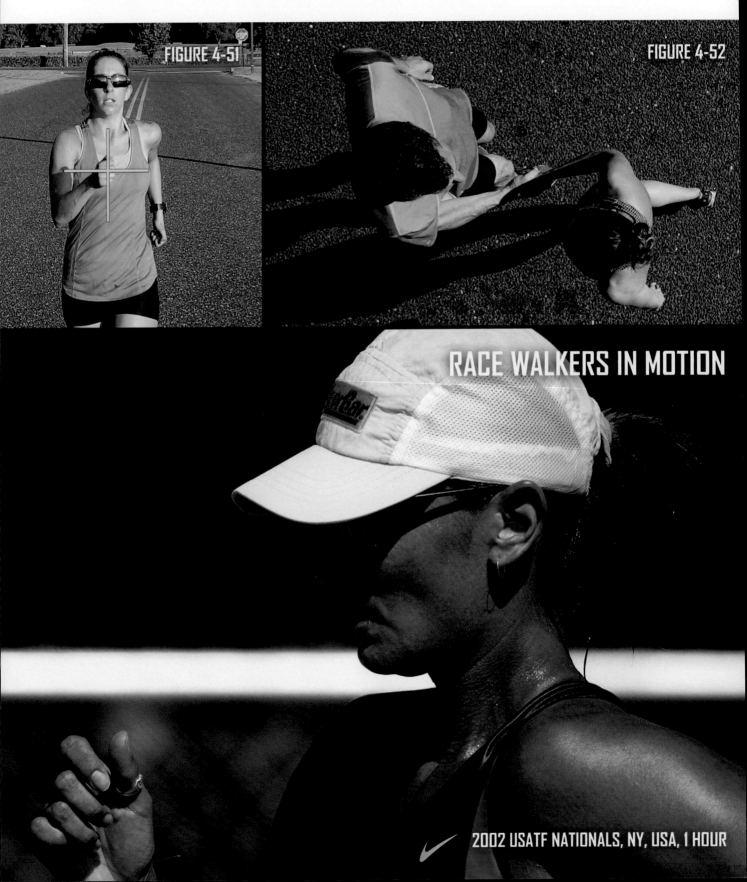

FIGURE 4-51

FIGURE 4-52

RACE WALKERS IN MOTION

2002 USATF NATIONALS, NY, USA, 1 HOUR

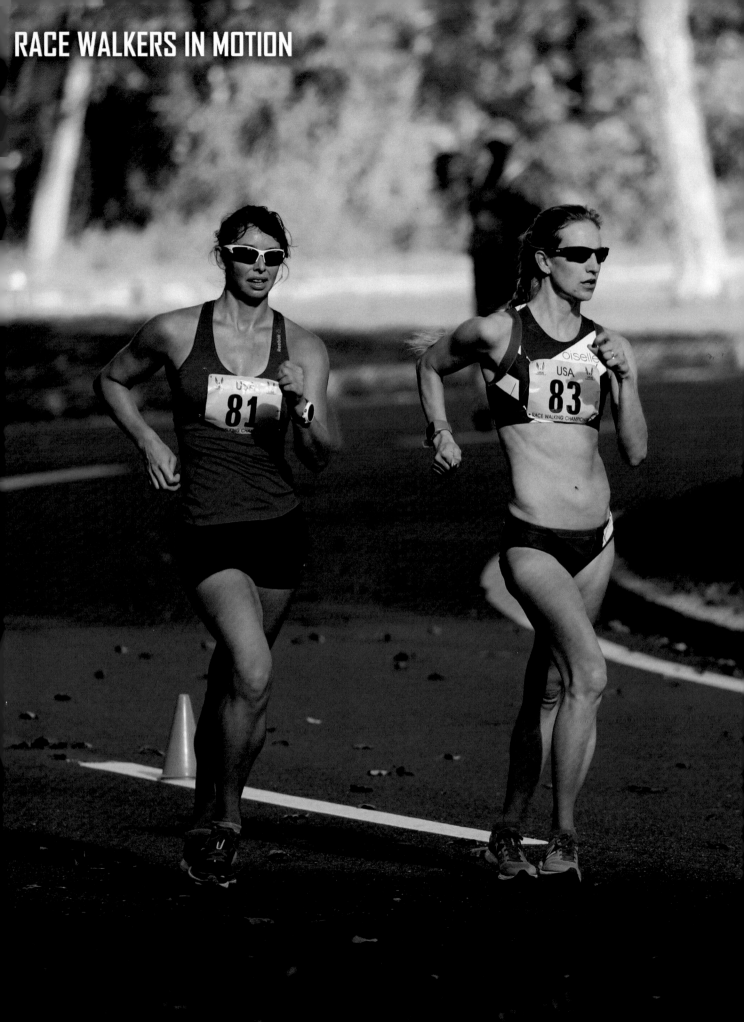

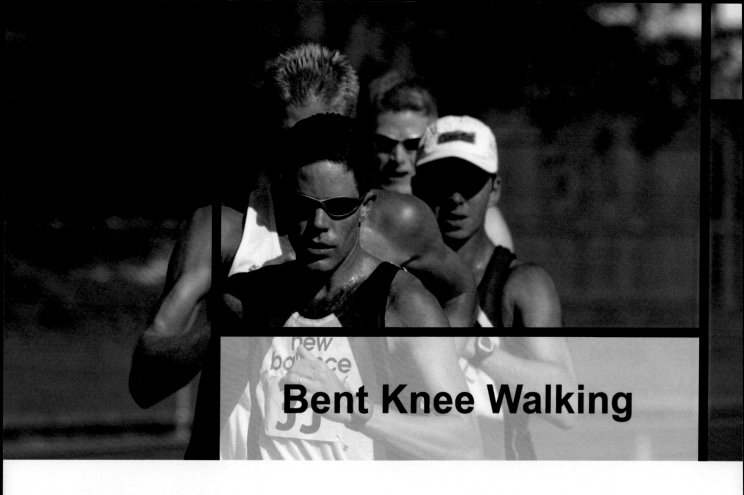

Bent Knee Walking

According to international judge Ron Daniel, 25 percent of all judges' calls in elite races are for bent knees. In searching through 8,000 photos from Olympic and World Cup race walks we found only 2 instances of bent-knee race walking (Figure 5-1). While there may be more cases that the camera didn't capture, the lack of photographic evidence is alarming.

Of the elites who were bent-kneed, one case was at a water stop and the other around a turn.

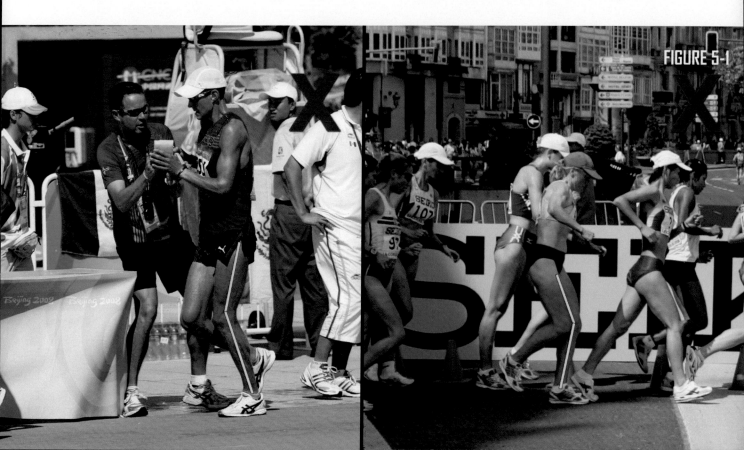

FIGURE 5-1

The story is different with masters race walkers and beginners. People come to race walking from a variety of backgrounds, but virtually none of them require, in daily life, that they walk with a straightened knee or the toe pointed as it is at a race walker's heel strike. Therefore, at first, straightening the knee at heel strike and maintaining a straightened knee until the leg passes under the body may prove difficult.

Let's review what the knee looks like when a race walker (Figure 5-2 through 5-4) is demonstrating proper race walking technique. The race walker's leg straightens simultaneously with the heel striking the ground. Then as the walker progresses forward, the leg stays straightened until it is in the vertical position and even beyond.

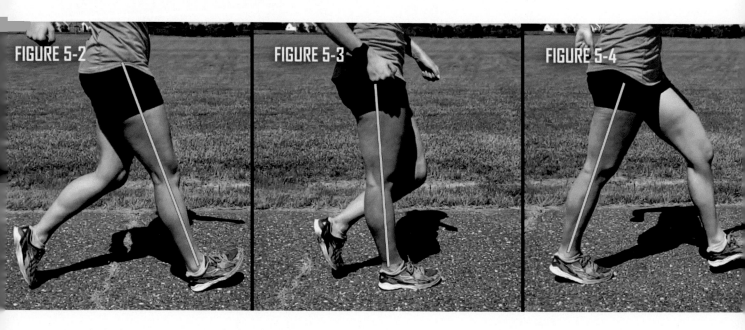

FIGURE 5-2   FIGURE 5-3   FIGURE 5-4

Now let's contrast the legal walker with a walker (Figure 5-5 to Figure 5-7) that isn't legal. Walkers that bend their knee come in many varieties. This walker never straightens his knee. Look how they land bent, never having achieved a full extension of the leg. The leg stays bent at the knee as the body's weight travels over it. Cases like this are easy to discern.

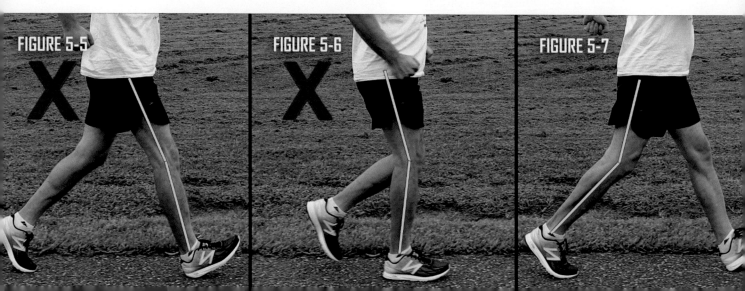

FIGURE 5-5   FIGURE 5-6   FIGURE 5-7

However, let's look at a subtler case. This walker lands with a fully extended, straightened leg (Figure 5-8), but as their weight travels over the leg, the knee bends (Figure 5-9 & 5-10) and the walker violates the definition of race walking.

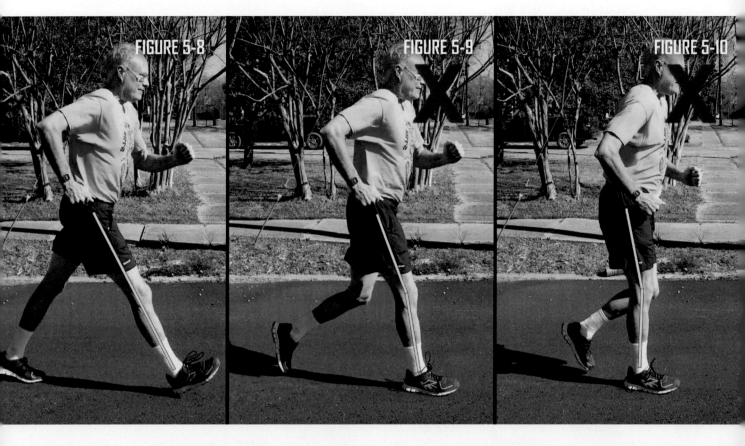

Sometimes walkers land without fully extending their lower leg at the moment the forward heel makes contact with the ground (Figure 5-11), but as they continue to progress through the stride (Figures 5-12 & 5-13) their leg straightens. This is also a violation of the definition of race walking.

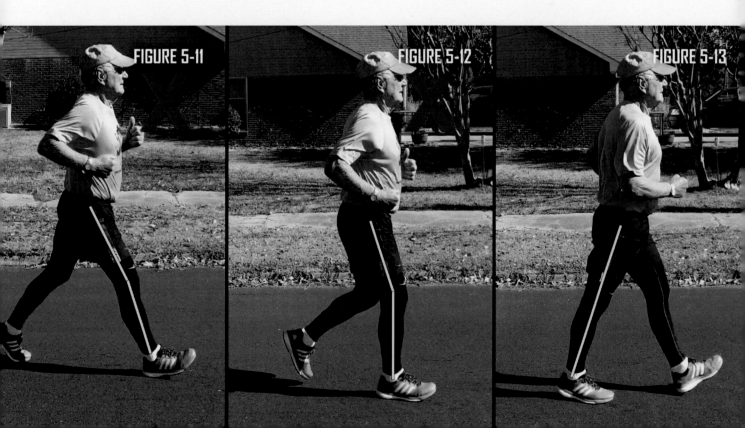

It takes a while to train the knee to maintain a straightened leg.

Don't despair; there are many corrective actions you can take to straighten up! Your first action should be your **focus**. There are a few key aspects of the stride, that when concentrated on properly, help a walker land fully extended and remain in the straightened position until the leg is at least past the vertical position.

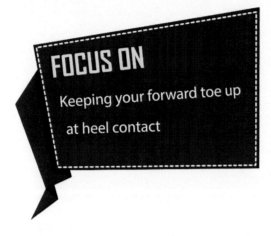

FOCUS ON

Keeping your forward toe up at heel contact

Try landing flatfooted and keeping your leg straightened as your weight is supported by the leg. It's not easy to do, especially if your foot lands any reasonable distance in front of your torso. See Figures 5-14 through 5-16 where the walker never points his toes off the ground. This is an obvious violation of the definition of race walking.

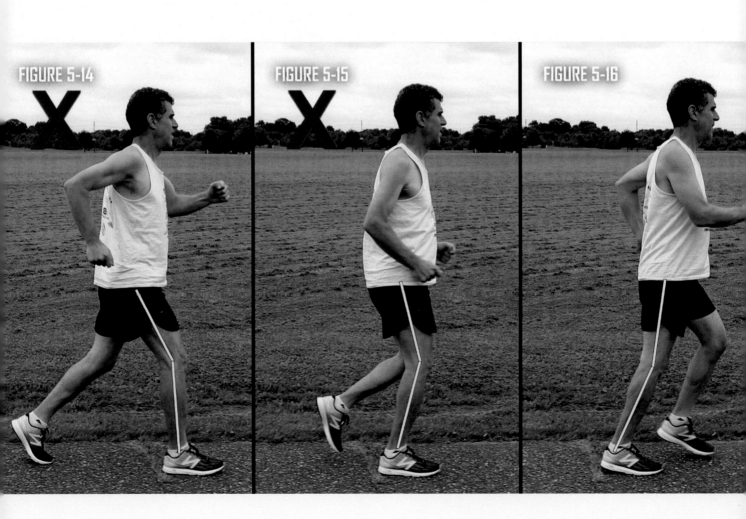

FIGURE 5-14   FIGURE 5-15   FIGURE 5-16

While most people do not land flatfooted when they race walk, you may be like many who land with the toe pointed (Figure 5-17), but then flatten the foot too quickly (Figure 5-18). Therefore, try to focus on keeping the toes of your foot pointed up as your heel strikes the ground (Figure 5-19). Then, as your torso comes forward over the supporting leg, roll through the foot, gradually lowering the toes to a flatfooted position (Figure 5-20). Notice the angle of the leg in Figure 5-18 vs 5-20. While the walker in Figure 5-20 if further along in his stride, his toes are higher off the ground than the walker in Figure 5-18. A simple check is to listen for your toes slapping into the ground. If you hear them, you are not holding them up long enough.

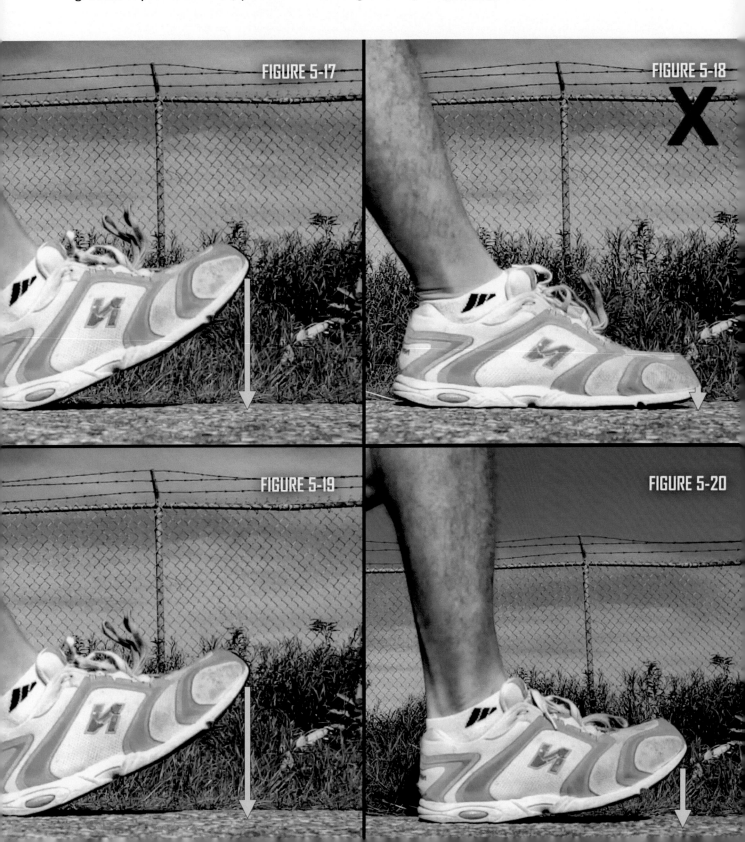

FIGURE 5-17

FIGURE 5-18

FIGURE 5-19

FIGURE 5-20

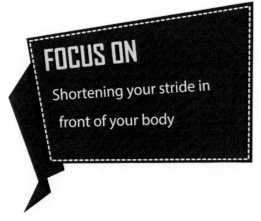

Bent-knee walking is often caused by striking the ground too far in front of the body. If you are over striding while you walk, you may land with a straightened knee (Figure 5-21).

However, as your torso moves forward, the bulk of your body's weight is loaded onto the supporting leg and the knee begins to bend (Figure 5-22 & 5-23). As it does, the quadriceps muscles fire, attempting to straighten your leg.

If you focus on a shorter stride in front of your body, your leg supports less weight and it is easier for you to keep the knee straightened.

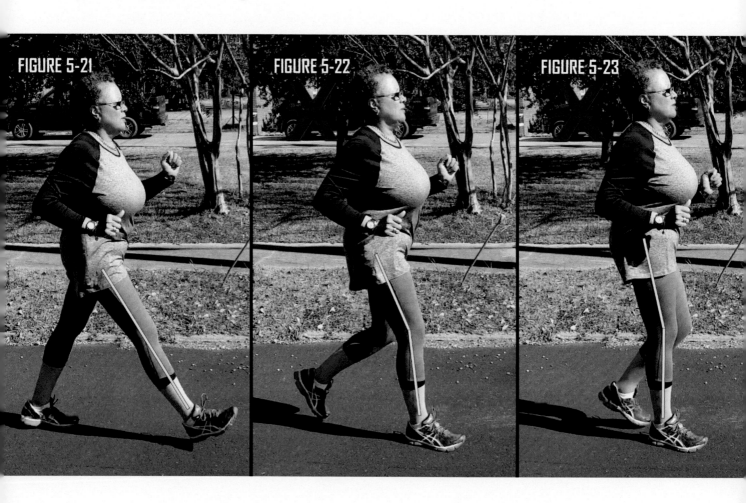

FIGURE 5-21   FIGURE 5-22   FIGURE 5-23

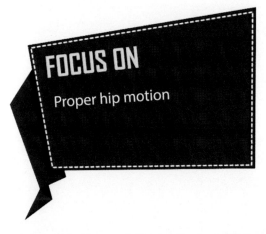
You can also improve the ratio of the step by focusing on proper hip rotation. Observe the effect of underutilizing your hips (Figure 5-24) when contrasted with the same walker simply focusing on driving their hip forward (Figure 5-25). When utilizing more forward hip drive, the walker shifts the ratio of the stride so that even more of their stride is behind their body.

In addition, notice how in Figure 5-25 the walker rolls onto their toes when the foot strikes the ground. This reduces the braking force caused the foot making contact in front of the body. In addition`n to improving efficiency, it also helps with correcting bent knee because less of the step is in front of the body and thus you reduce the time needed to hold the leg in the straightened position.

Finally, while not directly related to correcting bent knee, it's worth noting that modest improvement in forward hip rotation in this example increases the step length by almost two inches.

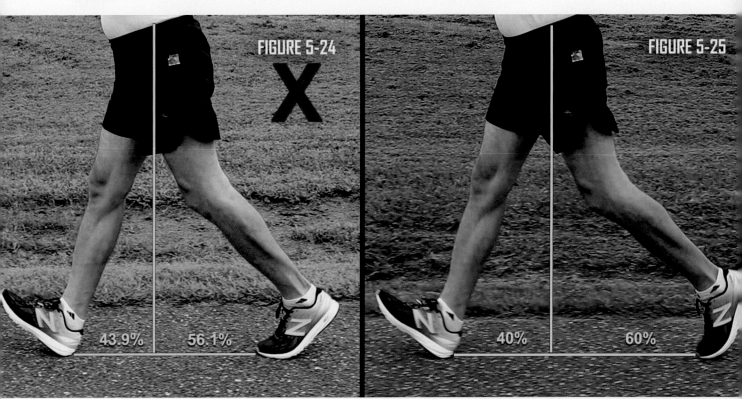

FIGURE 5-24   FIGURE 5-25

43.9%   56.1%   40%   60%

However, focus alone doesn't usually solve the problem. Strengthening the muscles used to straighten the leg and improving the flexibility of your hips, hamstrings, shins, and calves greatly assist walking with proper legal technique. Therefore, you should include the following exercises and stretches before your workouts.

ISOMETRIC KNEE EXERCISE

The **Isometric Knee** exercise is a mild strength training exercise that requires no extra weight and minimal movement of your body. It's isometric (using tension without contraction) and trains your muscle memory to know what it feels like to straighten the knee.

BODY POSITION

Sit down with your legs extended and a towel wrapped under your knees (Figure 5-26).

STEPS

A) Press down on the towel, straightening your knee (Figure 5-27). This causes your heels to lift off the ground.
B) Hold for 3 seconds.
C) Relax for 3 seconds. This causes your heels to return to the ground (Figure 5-26).
D) Repeat 10-15 times. This can be done one leg at a time or with both legs simultaneously.

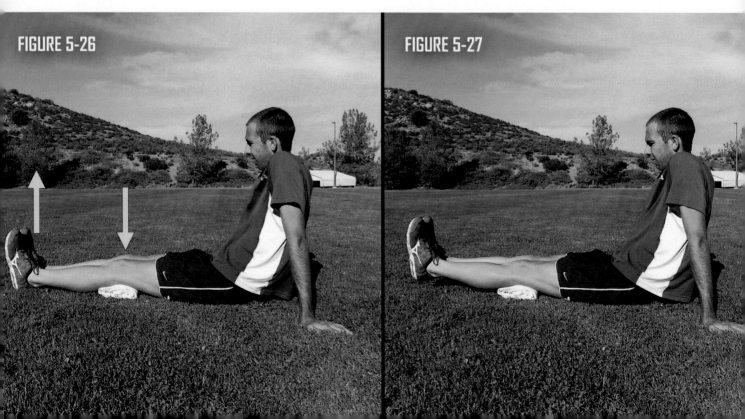

FIGURE 5-26

FIGURE 5-27

STRAIGHT LEG RAISE
EXERCISE

Like the isometric exercise shown earlier, this **Straight Leg Raise** exercise strengthens the quadriceps, but it also strengthens the hip flexors and abdominals. Since it strengthens your leg while keeping it straightened, it helps to promote muscle memory that enables you to walk without bending your knees at the incorrect time.

BODY POSITION

This exercise can be done with or without a light ankle weight. It's best to start without weight and gradually add light weights, building up to but never exceeding 10 percent of your body weight.

Lay on your back and support your body by bending one leg (Figure 5-28).

STEPS

A) Slowly raise the other straightened leg to about 45 degrees (Figure 5-29); hold it there for a second, and then gradually lower it.
B) Repeat this exercise 15 times with one leg, then switch and repeat with the other leg.
C) Perform 3 sets.

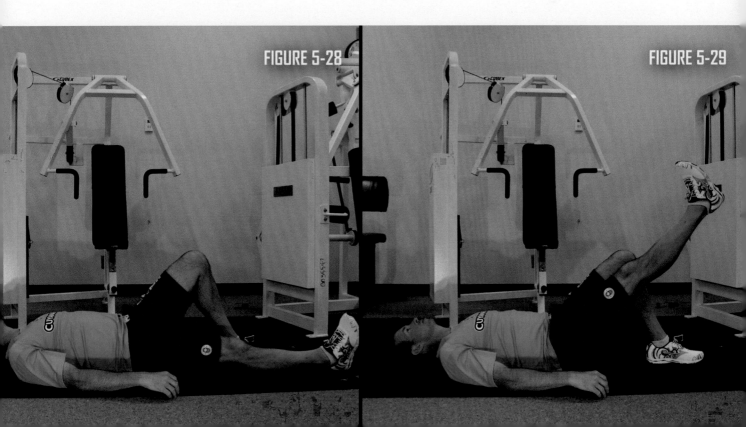

FIGURE 5-28   FIGURE 5-29

WRITE THE ALPHABET
EXERCISE

Writing an imaginary alphabet with your foot can strengthen and stretch the minor muscles around the ankle and can really help with your heel plant, roll through, and push off. When your lower leg muscles aren't strong enough, either you will land flatfooted or your foot will flatten very quickly. If your foot is flat on the ground while it is still in front of your torso, your risk of a bent knee call is high.

BODY POSITION

Sit down in a chair with one leg placed over the other.

STEPS

A) Slowly spell each capital letter of the alphabet with your toe (Figures 5-30 & 5-31).
B) Repeat with the other leg / foot.

OPTIONS

If you have a light ankle weight, you can place it around your foot and add extra resistance. This resistance could also be accomplished using an elastic band.

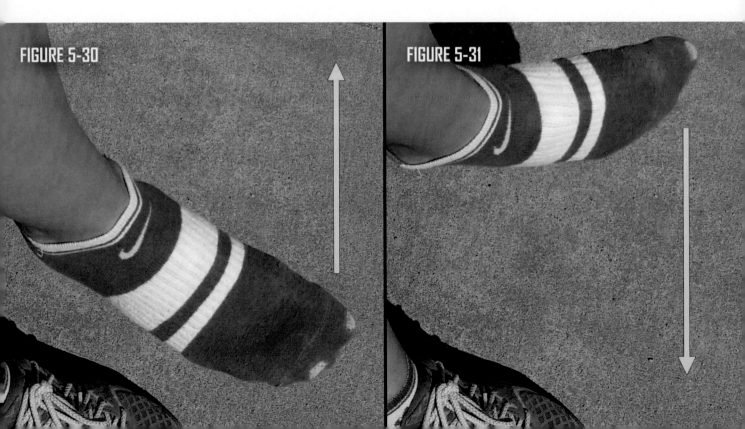

FIGURE 5-30

FIGURE 5-31

HEEL PLANT DRILL

The old adage of "take baby steps" is also true for race walking drills. Walking slowly with an exaggerated heel plant is a superb way to practice landing with a straightened knee without the pressure of going fast. This drill also allows you to develop the feel for proper foot roll.

BODY POSITION

Perform this drill using legal race walking technique.

STEPS

A) Start by taking a short step, emphasizing the toe up and straightened knee (Figure 5-32).
B) Roll through the stride, keeping the supporting foot's toes off the ground as long as possible.
C) Pick the foot up (Figure 5-33) and place the swing leg's foot down directly in front of the body (Figure 5-34), again emphasizing the toe up and straightened knee.
D) Repeat for 30 meters.

While performing this drill, you will feel all the small muscles of your foot working.

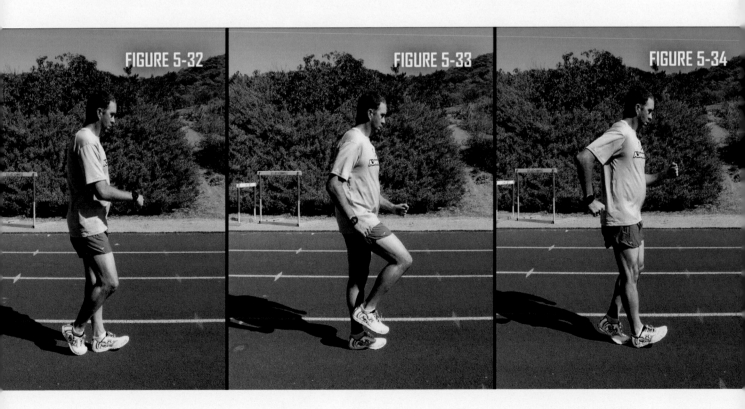

FIGURE 5-32   FIGURE 5-33   FIGURE 5-34

FOOT PLANT
DRILL

As explained in chapter 3, page 12 the *Foot Plant* drill can train your body to straighten your knee upon foot strike.

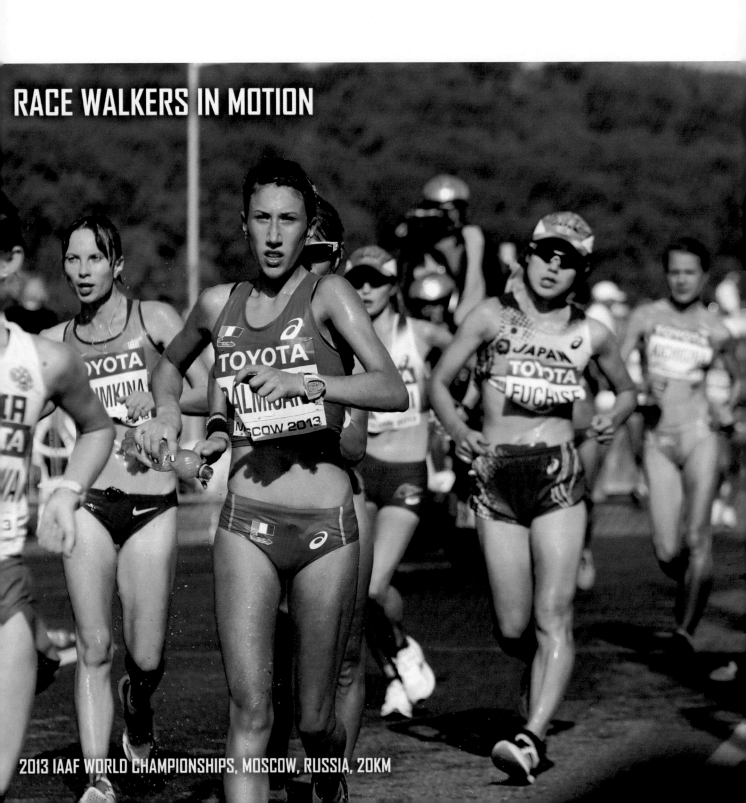

RACE WALKERS IN MOTION

2013 IAAF WORLD CHAMPIONSHIPS, MOSCOW, RUSSIA, 20KM

LONG STRIDES - LONG ARMS DRILL

An improvement in forward hip rotation is likely to improve your ability to straighten the knee on impact and keep it straightened until your leg passes the vertical position. When your hips rotate forward, the amount of your stride in front of your torso is reduced, thus reducing the likelihood that your leg bends as you ride forward on it. Therefore, the **Long Strides - Long Arms** drill and any other drills that target improved forward hip rotation are very useful to avoid bent-knee issues.

BODY POSITION

Perform this exercise while race walking.

STEPS

A) Keeping both arms straight and your hands flat with your palms back, race walk with an exaggerated stride by driving your hips forward (Figures 5-35 & 5-36).
B) Perform this exercise for 30 meters. You should feel a connection between your arms and hips.

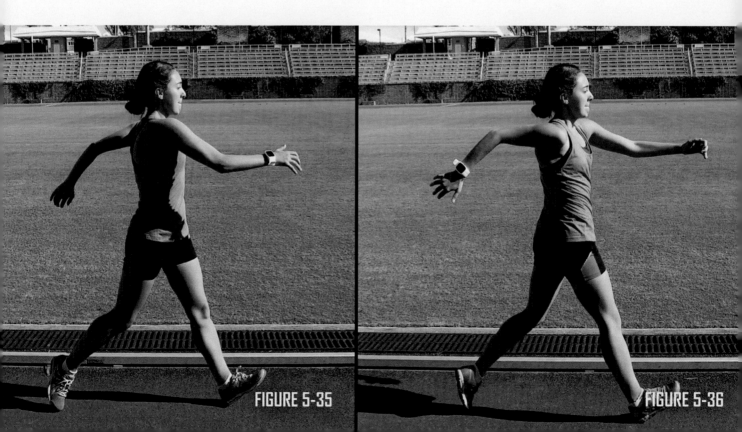

FIGURE 5-35

FIGURE 5-36

BEND DOWN HAMSTRING DRILL

The hamstrings are active during every phase of a race walker's stride. Sometimes they are eccentrically contracting (tensing the muscle as it lengthens); at other times they are concentrically contracted. Either way, it is imperative that we keep them flexible to maximize their efficiency and ensure that the leg can be straighten properly.

BODY POSITION

Standing straight up.

STEPS

A) Place one extended leg six inches in front of your body with toes pointed up.

B) Bend over slowly and, without bending the knee of your extended leg, reach to touch your toes (Figure 5-37).

C) Walk forward, alternating legs and if you are flexible, try reaching beyond your toes (Figures 5-38 & 5-39).

D) To relieve the stress on your back, make sure your buttocks is behind your rear foot when touching your toes.

E) Perform this exercise for 30 meters.

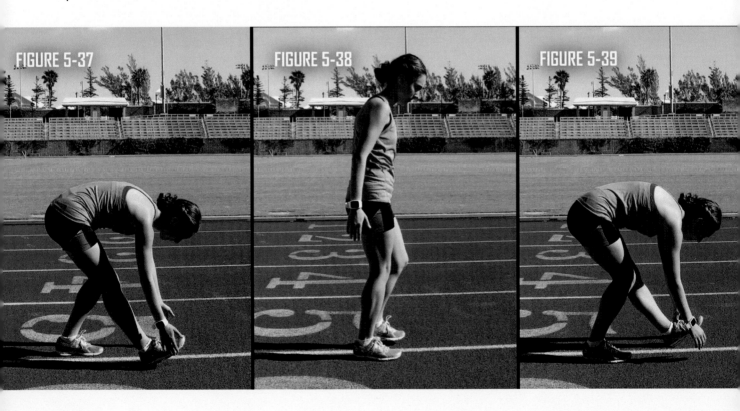

FIGURE 5-37   FIGURE 5-38   FIGURE 5-39

WALK ON HEELS
DRILL

One of the biggest physical causes of bent-knee walking is a lack of adequate shin strength to allow the foot to land with the toe pointed and properly roll through toe off. The single easiest way to strengthen your shins is to walk on your heels.

BODY POSITION

Standing straight up.

STEPS

A) Walk slowly, with a stride of no more than six inches (Figures 5-40 through 5-42). Remember, it's not a race.
B) Focus on how high you point your toes. The higher you point them, the better and more intensely you work your shins.
C) Maintain this technique for 30 meters.

TAKE CARE!!!

If your shins can't handle this distance, stop walking on your heels briefly and stretch out your shins (See chapter 5, page 61). Once you have stretched properly, resume heel-walking the remainder of the 30 meters. Upon completion, always stretch out the shins completely. You'll feel much happier that you did.

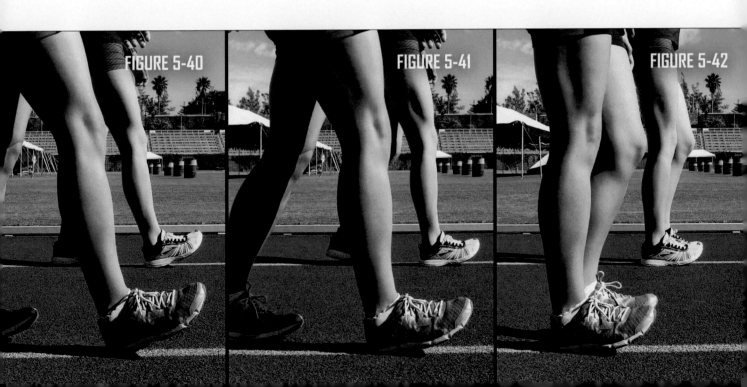

FIGURE 5-40 FIGURE 5-41 FIGURE 5-42

TOE RAISE
EXERCISE

The *Toe Raise* exercise is another good shin strengthening activity to help you land with your toe pointed and roll through to toe off.

BODY POSITION

Perform this more advanced shin exercise on the edge of a curb or step. Because balance is sometimes difficult when performing this exercise, make sure that you have a pole, wall, or anything to steady yourself. Facing away from the curb/step, place your heels as close to the edge as possible, taking care to remain steady.

STEPS

A) Pump your toes up and down as quickly as possible while maintaining balance and form (Figures 5-43 through 5-44).
B) Focus on getting your toes up high and low. The greater the range of motion your toes pass through, the better the workout. Upon completion, always stretch out the shins.

TAKE CARE!!!

Please be cautious. The shin muscles are very small and easily irritated. If you overdo this exercise, the shin muscles will become tight and fatigued, making it difficult to race walk properly.

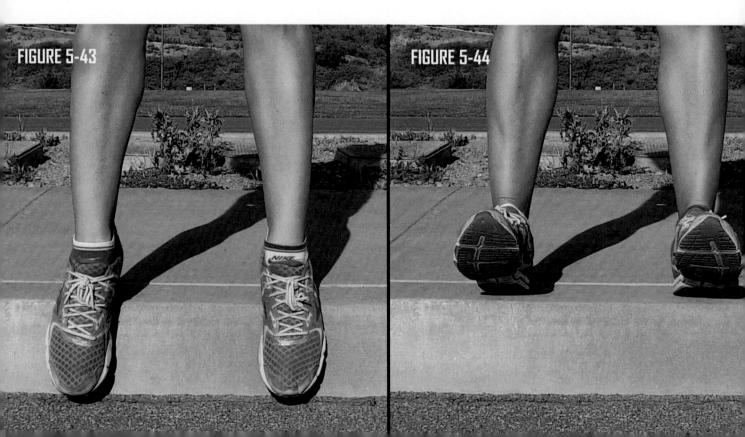

FIGURE 5-43

FIGURE 5-44

WALKING ON YOUR TOES
DRILL

Strengthening muscles involves balance. While athletes often focus on their shins to correct bent-knee walking, they neglect their complementary muscles, the calves. This exercise is similar to the shin strengthening exercise **Walk on Your Heels**. However, by slowly walking on your toes, you strengthen your calves.

BODY POSITION

Stand with your heels lifted off the ground.

STEPS

A) Walk slowly, it's not a race, with a stride of no more than six inches.
B) As you walk, focus on keeping your heels as high off the ground as possible (Figures 5-45 through 5-47).
C) Walk this way for about 30 meters.

TAKE CARE!!!

If your calves tire quickly, stop walking on your toes briefly and stretch your calves a bit (see chapter 5, page 57). Then complete the rest of the exercise. If walking 30 meters feels easy, try to go farther. The **Calf Raise** exercise also strengthens the calf muscles and help balance the shin strengthening exercises. In addition, by doing so, you enable yourself to push off more easily and with greater force.

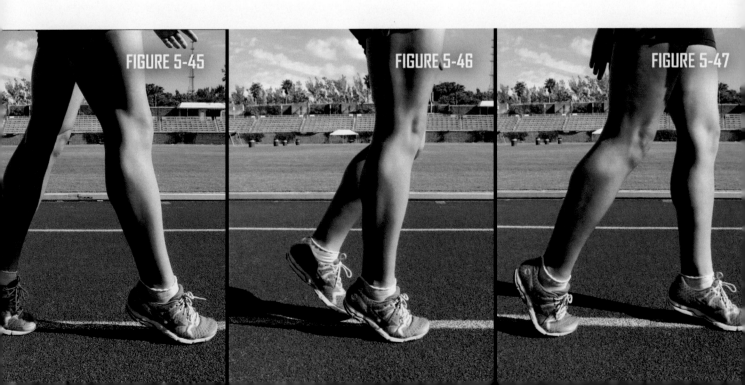

FIGURE 5-45   FIGURE 5-46   FIGURE 5-47

CALF RAISE
EXERCISE

This exercise is best executed with something nearby to help you maintain your balance. Ideally, practice the **Calf Raise** exercise on a curb near a pole or on a step with a handrail. Find a step or curb and position your toes as close to the edge as possible while still maintaining balance.

STEPS

A) Place both of your heels beyond the edge, raising and lowering them through a wide range of motion (Figures 5-48 & 5-49).

B) Repeat this motion 10 to 15 times, taking care not to cheat by using your upper body for leverage.

C) If you are strong enough, try raising and lowering your body on one foot at a time.

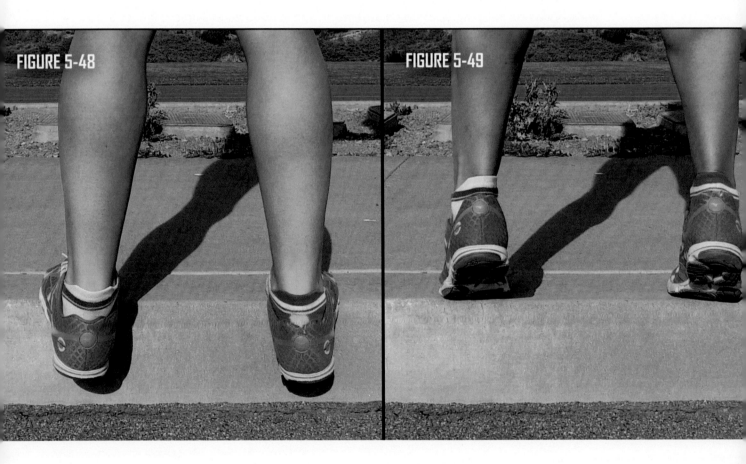

FIGURE 5-48

FIGURE 5-49

LEG EXTENSION WITH MACHINE
EXERCISE

Strong quadriceps are essential for race walking. The quadriceps help the lower leg to swing forward as quickly as possible and are directly responsible for helping to straighten the knee. The goal is to make them strong, but not too big, as large quadriceps hampers our efficiency. Therefore, we want to use low weights and a high number of repetitions to get the muscle in its optimal form for race walking.

BODY POSITION

Ideally, perform this exercise on a machine, one leg at a time. While machine models differ, most are similar in structure to the one shown. Higher-quality machines usually allow you to adjust the seat and leg roller. Set the equipment so that your knee is on the axis of the machine, with your ankle just below the leg roller.

STEPS

A) Keeping your shin pressed against the machine, extend your leg nearly to a locked position; exhale as you raise the bar (Figure 5-50).
B) While inhaling, lower your leg to its original position (Figure 5-51).
C) Repeat this exercise 20 times with each leg for 2-3 sets. As you execute the exercise, make sure that your ankle remains in contact with the roller and that you are controlling the weight.

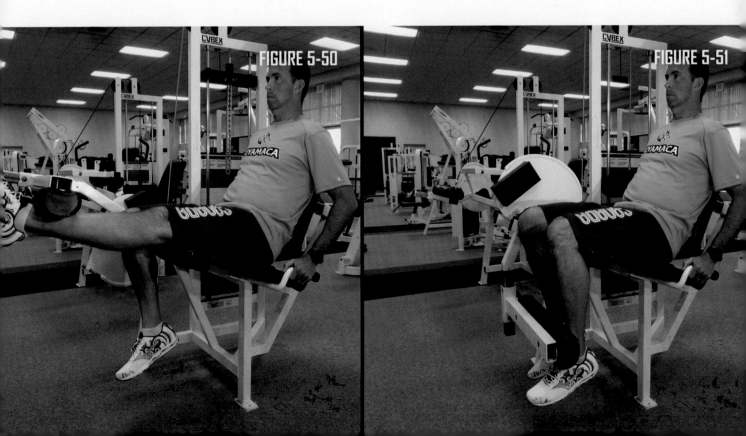

FIGURE 5-50 FIGURE 5-51

LEG EXTENSION WITHOUT MACHINE
EXERCISE

We know quadriceps strength is important, but some of us may not have a leg extension machine accessible. Here's a low-tech way to achieve the same results.

BODY POSITION

Sit in a tall stool or chair and strap a light ankle weight around your ankle; beginners may choose to skip the weight (Figure 5-52).

STEPS

A) Straighten the leg with the ankle weight (Figure 5-53).
B) While exhaling, lower the leg to the original position (Figure 5-52).
C) Repeat 15 times and then switch legs.
D) Repeat for 3 sets.

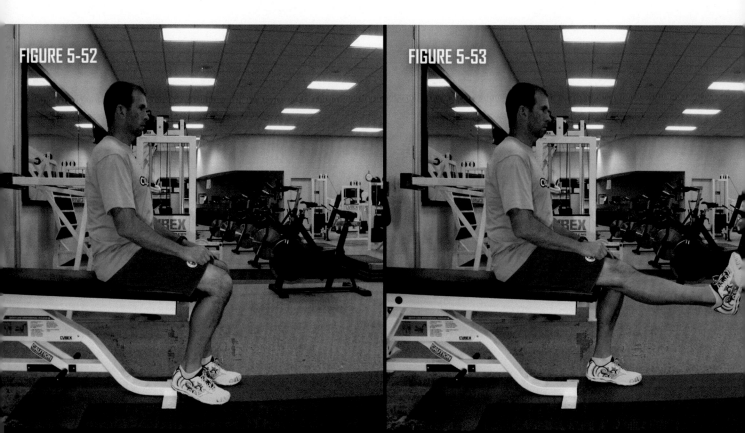

FIGURE 5-52

FIGURE 5-53

LEG CURL WITH MACHINE
EXERCISE

Strong hamstrings are important to race walking. The hamstrings are active during every phase of a race walker's stride. Sometimes they are eccentrically contracting; at other times they are concentrically contracted (tensing the muscle as it shortens). Either way, it is imperative that we keep them strong to maximize their efficiency and our legality.

BODY POSITION

This exercise is best performed on a machine, one leg at a time. With few exceptions, most machines are similar in structure to the one shown. Higher-quality equipment usually allows you to adjust the platform and leg roller; set them so that you situate your knee on the axis of the machine, with the ankle just below the leg roller (Figure 5-54).

STEPS

A) While exhaling and keeping your thigh pressed against the machine, curl your leg, pulling your heels inward so that the leg roller approaches your buttocks (Figure 5-55).
B) While inhaling, complete the exercise by lowering your leg back to its original position (Figure 5-54).
C) Always maintain contact between the roller and your leg as you execute the lift. Also pay attention to maintain control of the weight throughout the exercise.
D) Repeat 20 times with each leg and complete 3 sets.

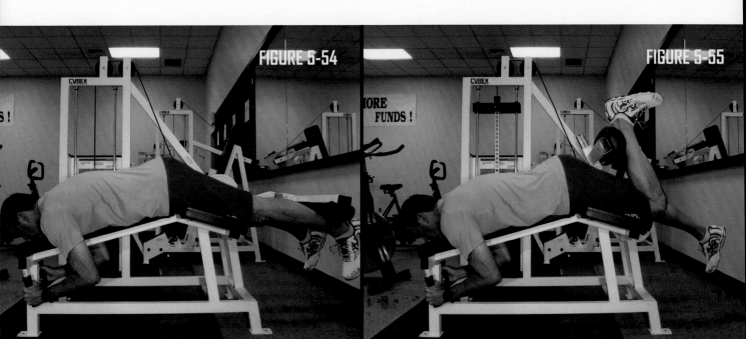

FIGURE 5-54   FIGURE 5-55

LEG CURL WITHOUT MACHINE
EXERCISE

We know hamstring strength is important, but some of us may not have a leg curl machine accessible. Here's a low-tech way to achieve the same results using an ankle weight to simulate the machine.

BODY POSITION

Either stand next to a wall / pole for balance or perform this exercise laying on a bench. Strap a light ankle weight around your ankle; beginners may choose to skip the weight (Figure 5-56).

STEPS

A) Raise the leg with the ankle weight, while inhaling, until your lower leg is parallel with the floor. Support yourself with the opposite leg (Figure 5-57).
B) Hold for one second.
C) Lower the leg, while exhaling, to the original position (Figure 5-56).
D) Repeat 20 times and then switch legs.
E) Repeat for 3 sets.

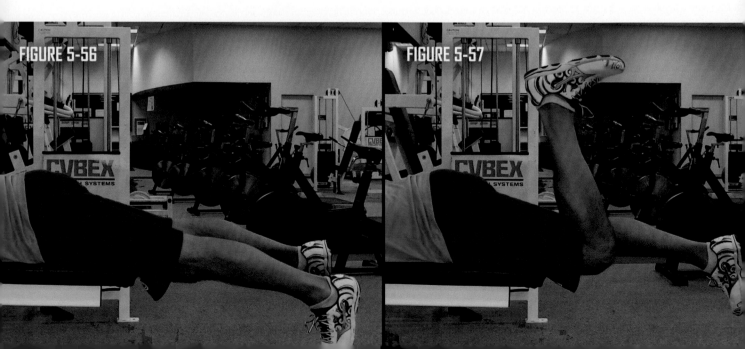

FIGURE 5-56

FIGURE 5-57

TRADITIONAL CALF STRETCH

If your calves are tight, it is difficult to point your toe and straighten your knee at heel strike. The *Traditional Calf* stretch is a great place to start and easy to do.

BODY POSITION

Place both hands at shoulder height on a wall or pole in front of your body. Keep your arms fairly straight and your lead leg bent under your body.

STEPS

A) Place the heel of your rear leg 1½ to 2 feet behind your body.
B) Keeping your rear leg fairly straight but not locked in position, place the heel of this foot on the ground (Figure 5-58 & 5-59).
C) You should feel a stretch down the outer part of your rear-leg calf muscle. If you don't, try moving your rear foot back a little farther (remember to place your heel back on the ground after you move your foot back).
D) Throughout the stretch, your upper body should remain vertical and straight; do not bend forward.
E) Alternate legs when finished.

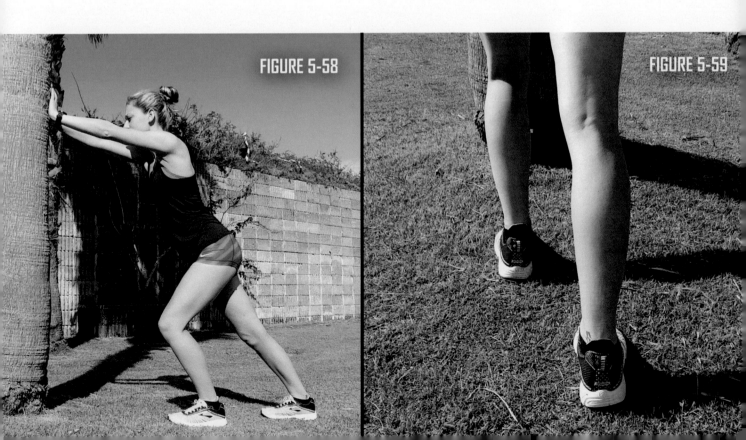

FIGURE 5-58

FIGURE 5-59

BENT KNEE CALF STRETCH

The calf is not a single muscle; it comprises two muscles, both of which need stretching. The previous stretch worked the outer calf muscle. The **Bent Knee Calf** stretch may not feel effective initially, but it utilizes an excellent position that stretches deep in the inner calf muscle (soleus).

BODY POSITION

You can start this stretch as you finish the *Traditional Calf Stretch*. (Figure 5-60)

STEPS

A) Place both hands, shoulder high, on a pole or wall in front of your body.
B) Keep your arms fairly straight with one leg slightly bent under your body.
C) Place the heel of your rear leg 1 to 1 ½ feet behind your body. Notice that this is about six inches in front of the placement for the *Traditional Calf Stretch*.
D) Keeping your rear leg fairly straight and in a stable position, place the heel of your rear foot on the ground (Figure 5-61).
E) Now, keeping your heel planted, bend the rear leg so that your knee drops a few inches closer to the ground.

You should feel a deeper but less pronounced stretch in your calf muscle. While not as pronounced as the other stretches, this one definitely works on the targeted muscle.

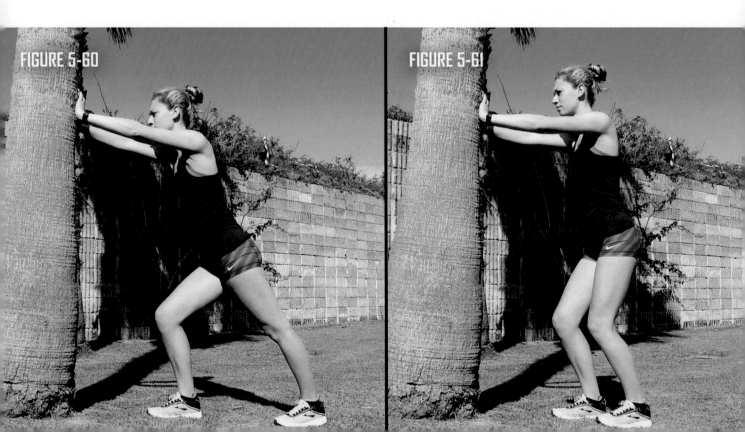

FIGURE 5-60

FIGURE 5-61

ADVANCED CALF
STRETCH

If your calves are extremely flexible, you may want a deeper more advanced calf stretch. Because this stretch is relatively aggressive, you may need to build up to it by practicing the *Traditional Calf* and *Bent Knee Calf* stretches first. The more flexible your calf muscles are, the better foot plant and roll through you will achieve.

BODY POSITION

Place one foot as close as possible to the edge of a step or curb while maintaining good balance. If possible, use a tree, pole, or even another walker for balance.

STEPS

A) While keeping your rear leg as straight as possible, lower your heel over the curb as far as it will go comfortably (Figure 5-62). You'll achieve the best stretch by hanging as close to the edge as possible and lowering your heels as far as they will go.
B) After holding the stretch for 20-30 seconds, alternate legs.
C) If you still feel tight, repeat this stretch more than once.

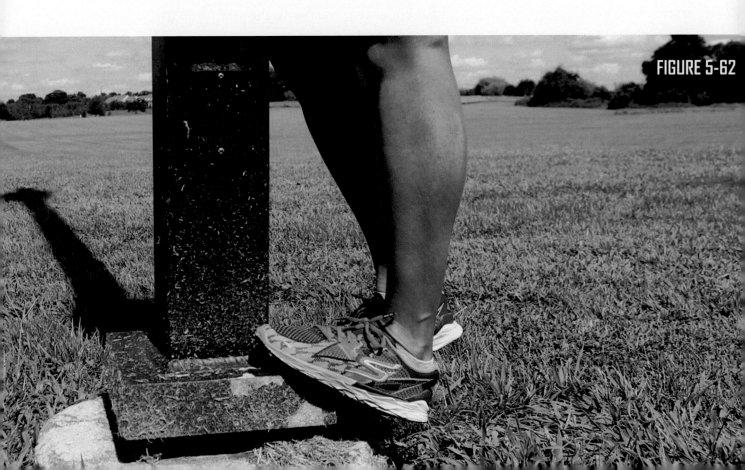

FIGURE 5-62

INTENSIVE CALF
STRETCH

The *Intensive Calf* stretch is the most aggressive calf stretch included. We use it to stretch the upper areas of the calf that are not reached by less intensive stretching. Definitely perform the other calf stretches before attempting this one.

BODY POSITION

Once again, you will need a wall, pole or tree for support. Begin by standing about an arm's length away from the pole (The closer to the pole you stand, the more you stretch the calf) with your pelvis forward (not bent at the waist).

STEPS

A) Place the heel of the first leg close to the bottom of the pole with the toes against it, as if you were trying to step on the pole.
B) Now keep your leg and back straight and lean into the wall slowly (Figures 5-63 & 5-64).
C) Being careful not to reach the point of pain, lean into your front leg until you feel moderate tension in your upper calf.
D) Hold the stretch for 20 to 30 seconds, then alternate legs.

Be sure to use care when first executing this stretch as you can easily overextend your calf if you bounce or move into this position too forcefully. Unlike the first two calf stretches, the advanced stretch concentrates on the muscles of your upper calf. You may want to work up to this position by practicing the other stretches for a few weeks first.

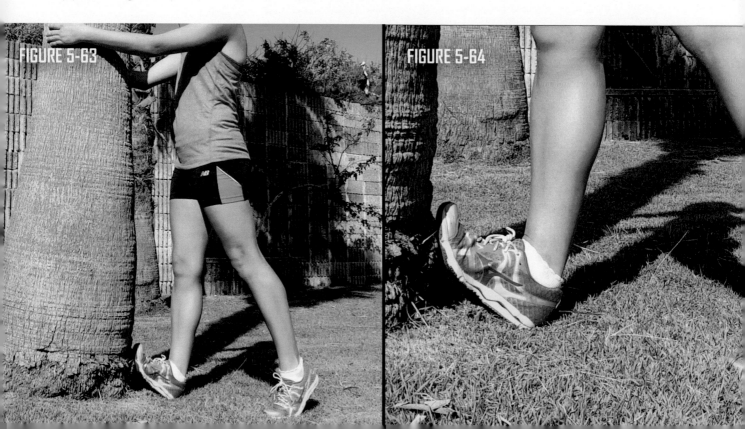

FIGURE 5-63

FIGURE 5-64

STANDING SHIN
STRETCH

All race walkers will tell you that their shins take a real beating from race walking, and when your shins are sore it becomes difficult to land with the toes pointed up. Therefore, we must treat our shins kindly. If you don't, you'll surely develop shin splits and know firsthand how this tiny little muscle can cause big problems. The **Standing Shin** stretch is just one way to take care of it. However, be careful not to overdo it; otherwise the shin muscle will get back at you on your next walk.

BODY POSITION

Balance yourself near a pole or wall. Put your weight on the supporting leg.

STEPS

A) Now touch the other foot to the ground, toe first, and pull your rear foot forward just to the point where it is about to move forward.

B) Hold it there (Figures 5-65 & 5-66); you should feel the shin muscles elongate and loosen up.

Do not rest on the bottom of the front of your foot as currently shown in Figure 5-67.

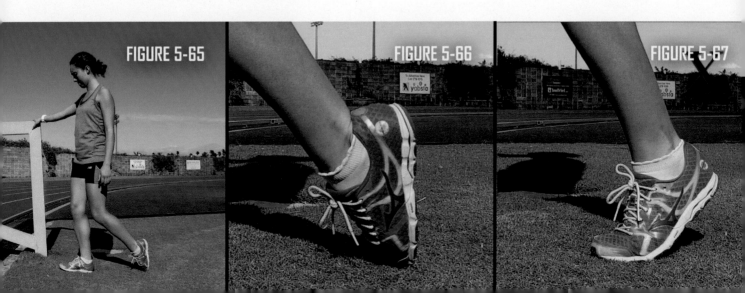

FIGURE 5-65
FIGURE 5-66
FIGURE 5-67

SEATED SHIN STRETCH

The **Seated Shin** stretch is an effective stretch but has drawbacks. For one thing, you must sit on the ground. If you are in the middle of a race, this is particularly inconvenient. The other problem is that you need grass to perform the stretch, or some very tough knees. Nevertheless, this stretch is very effective in loosening overworked shins and enables you to point your toe and roll through properly.

BODY POSITION

Sit on the grass or soft carpet with your legs folded directly under your thighs.

STEPS

A) See Figures 5-68 & 5-69; note that the shoelaces touch the ground.
B) Use one hand to support your weight and the other to lift your knee.
C) This lifting should send a stretch down your shin.
D) Hold it 20 to 30 seconds, and then switch legs.

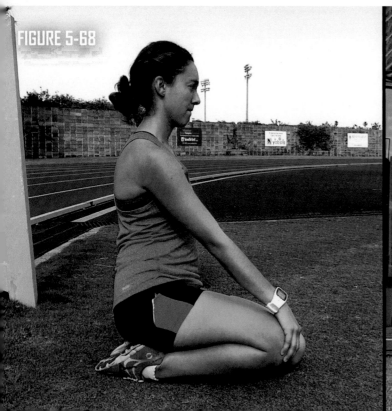

FIGURE 5-68

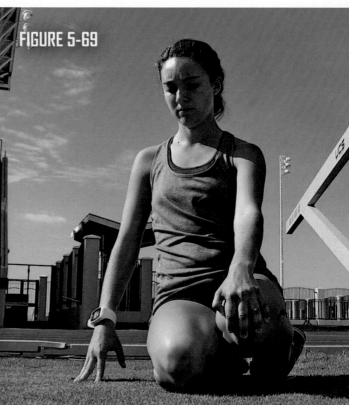

FIGURE 5-69

BACK OF THE KNEE
STRETCH

Sometimes a pain creeps up on you out of nowhere, as with pain behind the knee. Race walking sometimes aggravates this area, and it sneaks up so slowly that you don't actually realize it until it's too late. With a pain behind the knee, it is very difficult to straighten the knee properly. Avoid this potentially painful problem by adding the *Back of the Knee* stretch to your cool-down routine.

BODY POSITION

In a seated position, place one leg straight in front of you. Bend the knee of the non-stretching leg, placing the foot on the inside of the opposite thigh, forming a triangle.

STEPS

A) Keeping a straight back, bend from the hips and lean toward your toe (Figure 5-70).
B) If your hamstring flexibility allows, pull your toes towards your body.
C) If you lack flexibility in the hamstrings and are not able to reach your toes, use a towel or rope to extend your reach (Figure 5-71) and get cracking on those hamstrings!

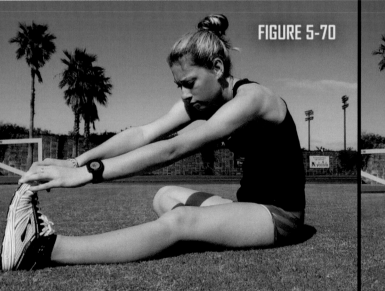
FIGURE 5-70

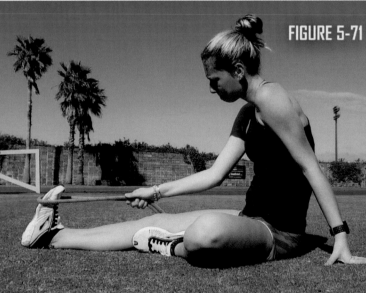
FIGURE 5-71

TRADITIONAL HAMSTRING STRETCH

Hamstring flexibility is a key to efficient race walking technique and is especially important for those walkers with bent knee issues. The simplest way to stretch your hamstrings is to perform the traditional hamstring stretch as either a cool down activity or after you've properly warmed up.

BODY POSITION

Sit down, placing one leg in front of you.

STEPS

A) Bend your other leg with the sole of your foot facing toward your straight leg and the knee pointed out.
B) Keeping your back straight, lean forward from the hips, reaching towards your toes (Figure 5-72).
C) Ideally, you should reach past your toes, but remember not to overstretch or bounce while trying to touch them; just stay within your comfort zone.
D) Hold the stretch for 20-30 seconds and repeat 2-3 times with each leg.

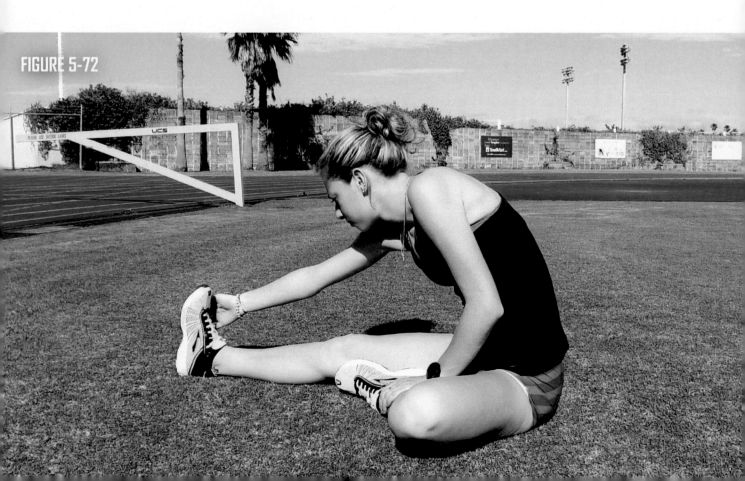

FIGURE 5-72

LEG UP HAMSTRING
STRETCH

Sometimes getting down on the ground to stretch your hamstring isn't very convenient. Instead, try stretching your hamstrings standing up using the *Leg Up Hamstring* stretch.

BODY POSITION

Place your foot on a bench, table, or anything at a comfortable height, while standing far enough back to straighten your leg comfortably.

STEPS

A) With a straight back, lean forward, taking care not to bend your knee.
B) Reach for the toes on your raised foot and hold once you begin to feel the stretch; You may also choose to hold behind your leg (Figure 5-73).
C) Hold the stretch for 20-30 seconds and repeat 2-3 times with each leg.

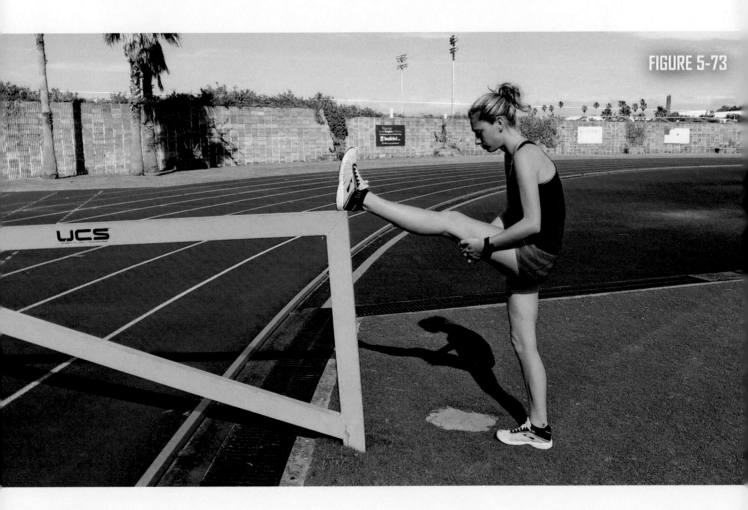

FIGURE 5-73

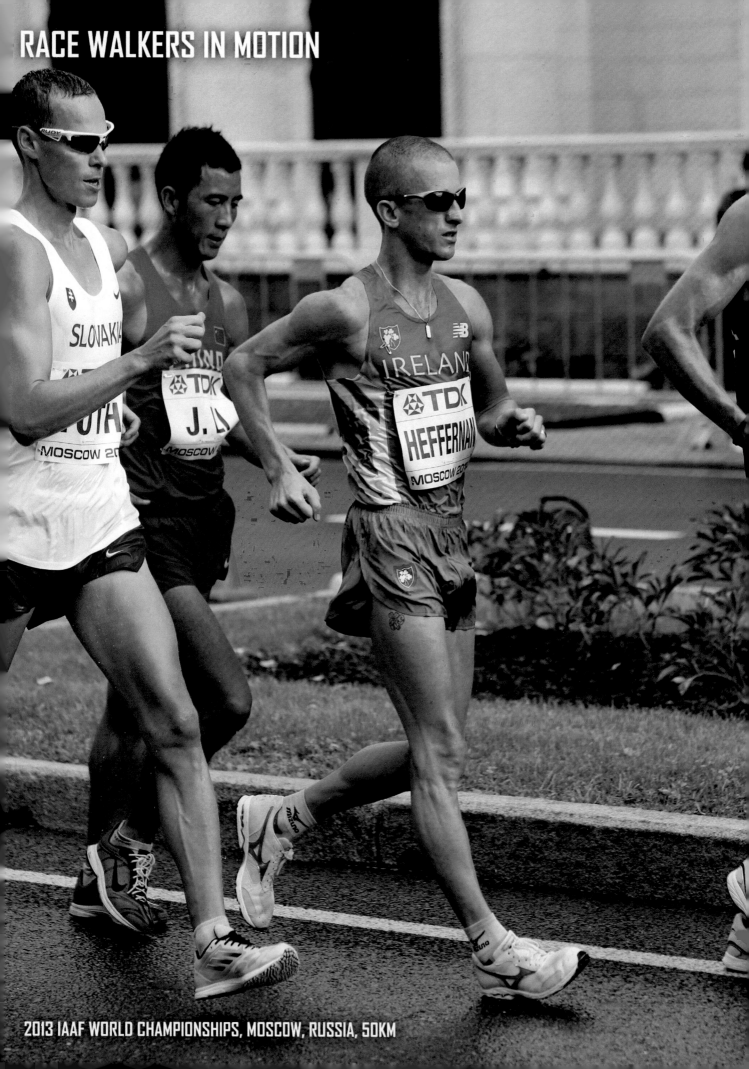

2013 IAAF WORLD CHAMPIONSHIPS, MOSCOW, RUSSIA, 50KM

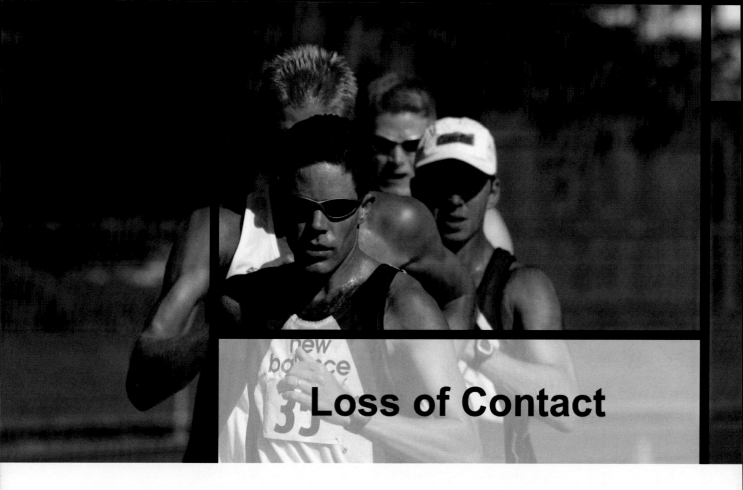

Loss of Contact

The definition of race walking has changed many times over the years. However, since the 1996 change in the definition of race walking, the determination of whether a race walker loses contact with the ground has become more subjective.

PRE 1996

WALKING IS A PROGRESSION BY STEPS SO TAKEN THAT UNBROKEN CONTACT WITH THE GROUND IS MAINTAINED AT EACH STEP, THE ADVANCING FOOT OF THE WALKER MUST MAKE CONTACT WITH THE GROUND BEFORE THE REAR FOOT LEAVES THE

1996 – PRESENT

RACE WALKING IS A PROGRESSION OF STEPS SO TAKEN THAT THE WALKER MAKES CONTACT WITH THE GROUND SO THAT NO VISIBLE (TO THE HUMAN EYE) LOSS OF CONTACT OCCURS

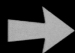
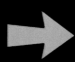

Because the definition now states that "the walker makes contact with the ground so that no visible (to the human eye) loss of contact occurs," it is now impossible to state quantitatively whether a race walker is in violation of the definition of loss of contact.

What one human eye perceives, another may not.

When a walker has a visible contact phase, which is significantly different than saying to look for a visible loss of contact, the answer is easily quantifiable. Let's look at these two walkers. The walker in Figure 6-1 has a pronounced double-support phase. When the swing leg's foot makes contact with the ground, the rear foot has not completed rolling up for toe-off. Instead, there is an extended period where both feet are in contact with the ground. This extended double-support phase allows a judge to easily discern a visible contact phase.

In contrast, if we look at the walker in Figure 6-2, whether there is a loss of contact is more difficult to discern with the human eye. She still has a moment of double contact, but it is only for an instant. Notice she has rolled up onto her toes at the moment the forward foot contacts the ground. This makes it difficult for a judge to observe accurately whether the walker has a visible contact phase in their stride.

A qualified judge should still be capable of identifying these walkers as they conform to the definition of race walking whether using the definition from before 1996 or the current definition. This is because with the new definition, the judge is not looking for visible contact but a visible loss of contact.

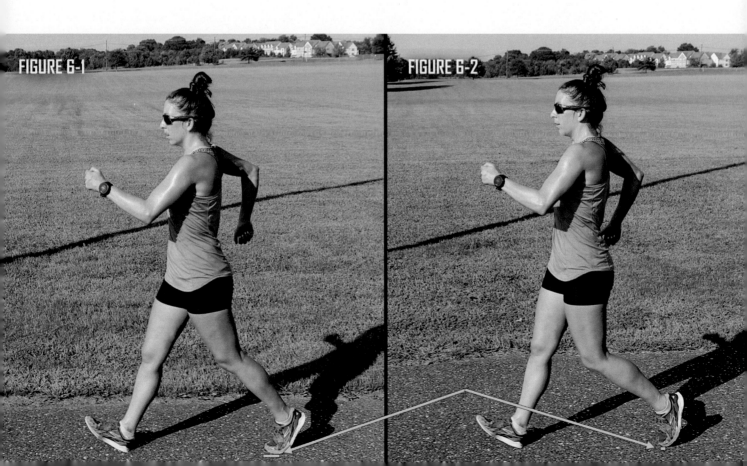

FIGURE 6-1   FIGURE 6-2

However, the decision of legality becomes blurrier as a race walker's stride contains a miniscule loss of contact phase. Through high speed videography, we can easily estimate the flight phase of a walker. The walker shown was shot using a camera capturing 240 frames per second (fps). That means for each frame the walker does not have contact with the ground, their estimated flight time of increases .0041 seconds.

In the old days, when video was recorded on tape, it was recorded at 24-30 frames per second. Therefore, having no contact with the ground for more than 1 frame and less than 2 frames approximated to being off the ground for about .033 seconds and that was considered the threshold for the human eye being able to discern that a person was off the ground. That estimate was subjective. If we use it as a barometer, somewhere between 7 to 8 frames of flight with a 240 fps camera is probably not detectable by the human eye.

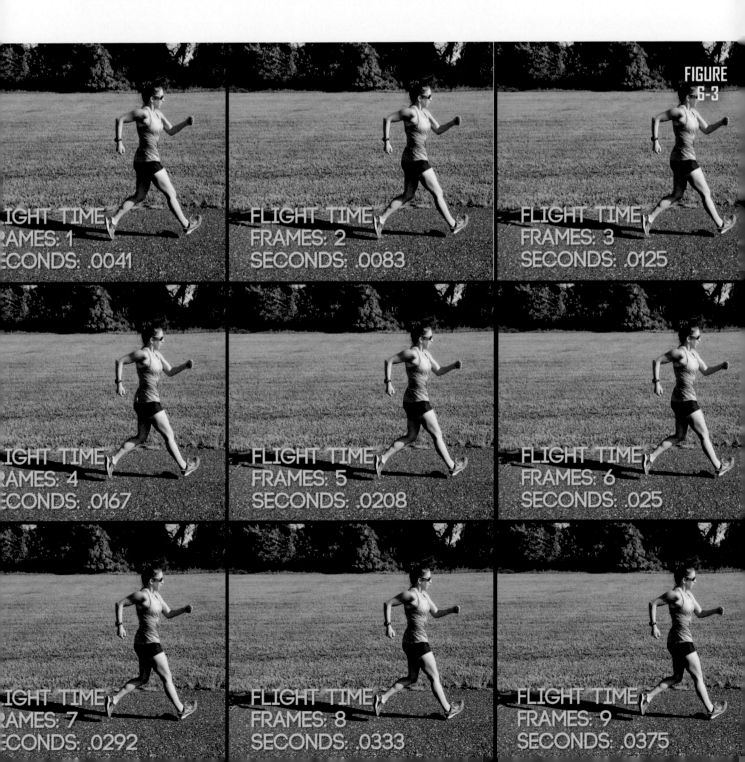

FIGURE 6-3

FLIGHT TIME
FRAMES: 1
SECONDS: .0041

FLIGHT TIME
FRAMES: 2
SECONDS: .0083

FLIGHT TIME
FRAMES: 3
SECONDS: .0125

FLIGHT TIME
FRAMES: 4
SECONDS: .0167

FLIGHT TIME
FRAMES: 5
SECONDS: .0208

FLIGHT TIME
FRAMES: 6
SECONDS: .025

FLIGHT TIME
FRAMES: 7
SECONDS: .0292

FLIGHT TIME
FRAMES: 8
SECONDS: .0333

FLIGHT TIME
FRAMES: 9
SECONDS: .0375

First, let's observe walkers with varying flight times. While it's not fair to judge from a still photo, we can still have an objective conversation about the following three images.

The walker in Figure 6-4 is barely off the ground. While there is a flight phase visible to the camera, it's not noticeable to even the keenest human eye. The walker in Figure 6-5 has lost contact for 4-5 frames. While an individual judge's optical acuity varies, it's probably safe to say that this would not be noticeable by the human eye. The walker in Figure 6-6 is off the ground by more than 8 frames. So, she is closer to being deserving of being disqualified, but still may not be above the threshold to be seen by the human eye.

To some, this may seem excessively generous. Judges have a very difficult job and that's why in most cases it requires more than one judge to disqualify a walker.

In the presentation, *Kinematics of Elite Race Walking*, Brain Hanley studied race walkers at the 2008 World Cup. 30 20Km men's flight times were measured. While 3 had no visible flight phase, 15 had at least .02 seconds of loss of contact and 12 had a loss of contact for at least .04 seconds. These measurements were made with a 50 fps camera, so the athlete's flight times could be almost .02 seconds greater than measured. You might be questioning if .04 seconds is too generous. However, none of the walkers studied were disqualified. So, it may be that our estimate of .033 seconds is significantly less that what trained judges can detect.

If you are new to race walking, unless you come from a very athletic background, you probably won't be losing contact with the ground initially.

If you have concern, you can either enter a race and see how you do, or you can have someone video you with a high frame rate camera, even a smart phone, and count the frames. Just do it in really bright light to help the camera expose your feet clearly.

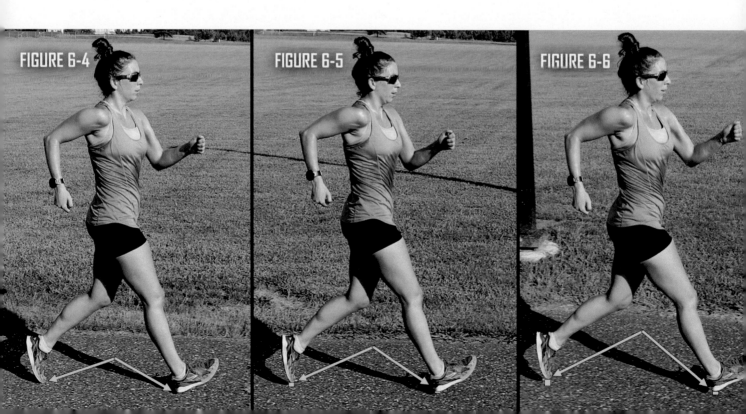

FIGURE 6-4 FIGURE 6-5 FIGURE 6-6

Correcting Loss of Contact

While it's easy to just say "slow down," there are many aspects of your stride that you can focus on instead of just slowing down.

If you can master these changes, then you might not have to slow down much, if at all, to reduce the perception that you are lifting.

While you may not be higher off the ground than the walker next to you, if you have excessive motion throughout your body you may draw the unwanted attention of judges.

Bouncing shoulders, bobbing heads, and arms flailing about are all unnecessary and inefficient. In addition to wasting energy, they can contribute to the perception that you are significantly off the ground. Judges should not determine if you are violating the definition based on excessive motion, but they may use it as a reason to observe you more closely.

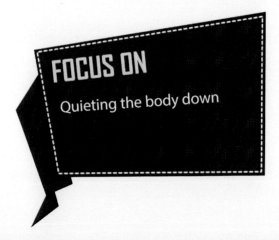

FOCUS ON

Quieting the body down

Focus on quieting your body. Try walking in front of a mirror on a treadmill while reducing excessive body motion. Focus on going forward, not up, down, or side to side. The instant feedback received by walking before a mirror goes a long way to improving your form.

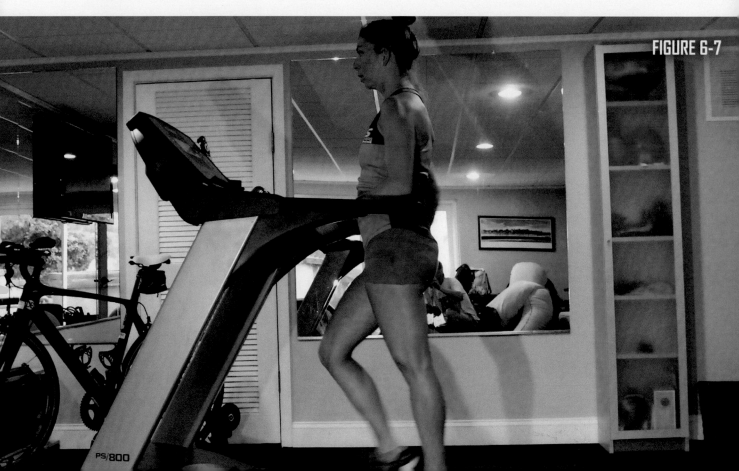

FIGURE 6-7

PS/800

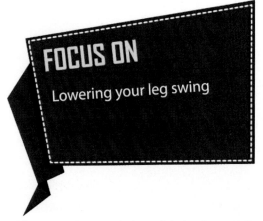

A big problem for walkers who get calls for lifting is the manner in which they carry their leg as it swings forward. A low foot and knee carriage as the leg swings forward is crucial to efficient technique. It is also pivotal to appearing legal.

Walkers who gallop forward, driving their knee high, inadvertently drive their foot forward higher off the ground. The difference may only be a matter of an inch or two, but that difference appears dramatic to a judge.

Observe Figures 6-8 and 6-9 where Miranda simulates a slight change in style by driving the knee higher. When we draw a horizontal line at heel height, we can see she is carrying her foot higher in Figure 6-8. We can also see other changes to her body position. She unconsciously leans forward and excessively increases the range of motion of her arms.

Focusing on a low vertical position of the foot and knee throughout the leg as it swings forward is one key to reducing your chance of a lifting call.

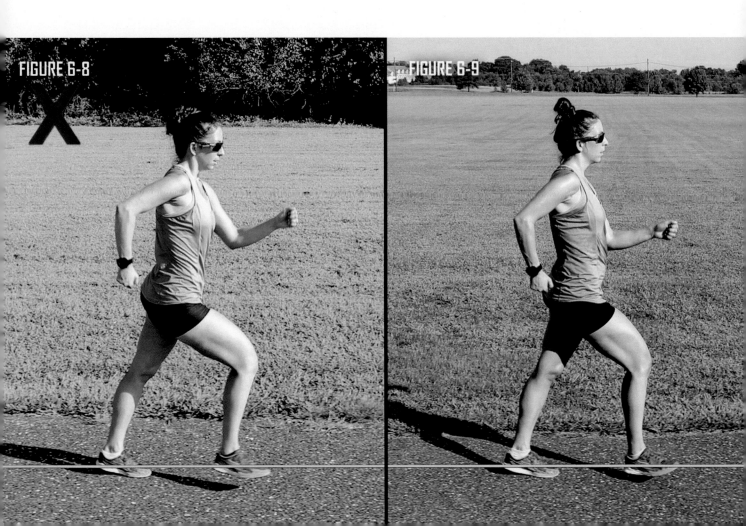

FIGURE 6-8

FIGURE 6-9

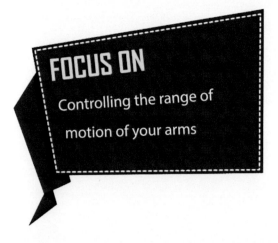

FOCUS ON

Controlling the range of motion of your arms

Overstriding in front of the body can also lead to lifting. When you reach out too far in front of your body, your foot hangs in the air, floating for all the judges to see. Often this is caused by swinging your arms too far in front of or behind your body.

Focus on good arm carriage and your legs should come back in line. Alternatively, lifting may be caused by reaching forward with your leg instead of your hips. Concentrate on placing the swing leg down shortly after it passes under the torso.

Observe how when Miranda overstrides in Figure 6-10 her leg is straightened, but she has neither placed her swing foot on the ground nor rolled up on the back foot. In contrast, in Figure 6-11, Miranda's swing foot strikes the ground simultaneously with her leg straightening and her rear foot rolling up onto it's toes. You can also observe that when she overstrides the angle that her leg extends from the body is greater, thus leading to an undesirable braking action.

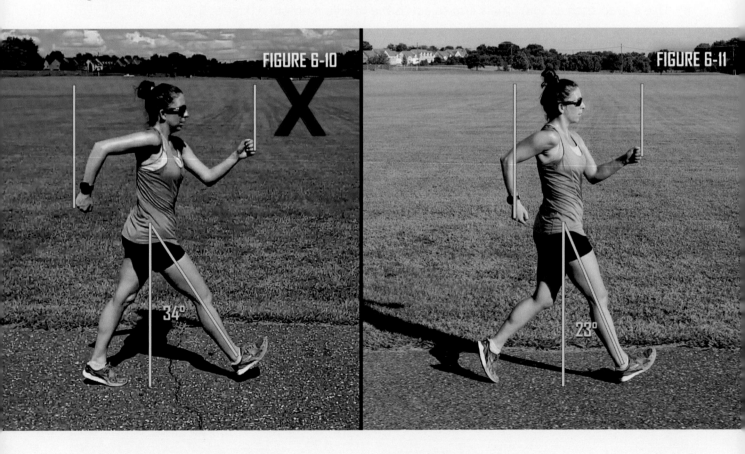

FIGURE 6-10

FIGURE 6-11

34°

23°

In addition to focusing on the key mental aspects causing lifting, you can also address the physical causes that lead to a visible flight phase. Two of the main offenders are a lack of hip flexor range of motion and tight hamstrings. Practicing the following exercises greatly improves your range of motion and assists in lengthening your stride behind your torso.

HURDLERS DRILL

The **Hurdlers** drill helps improve hip and groin flexibility while warming you up for race walking at the same time.

BODY POSITION

Lean against a wall or tree.

STEPS

A) While facing forward, swing your leg forward and up, then back and around, as if it were clearing a hurdle placed at your side (Figures 6-12 through 6-16).
B) Use a prop such as someone's arm to act as the hurdle if possible (Figure 6-17).
C) Range of motion is the key to performing this drill correctly; Be sure to extend your leg in as large a circle as possible by bringing your foot up as high as your knee on the swing through.
D) Perform this exercise 10-15 times for each leg.

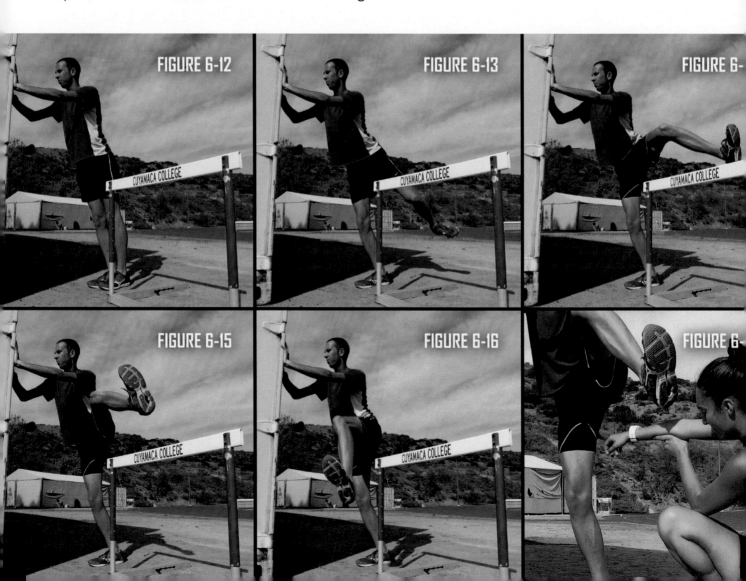

FIGURE 6-12   FIGURE 6-13   FIGURE 6-

FIGURE 6-15   FIGURE 6-16   FIGURE 6-

SIDE LEG SWING DRILL

Again, our mantra is that forward hip rotation is key to controlling lifting. Increasing the range of motion of your hips gives an athlete more time to get their swing foot down before the rear foot lifts off the ground.

The **Side Leg Swing** drill helps to improve hip and groin flexibility while warming you up for race walking at the same time.

BODY POSITION

Lean against a pole or tree.

STEPS

A) Swing your leg up and away from the body, kicking the leg as high as you can (Figure 6-18).
B) Swing the leg down and in front of the body, letting the hip move across the front of the body (Figure 6-19).
C) As the leg swings upward in front of your body, extend it as far as your range of motion allows (Figure 6-20).
D) You can lift the heel of your supporting leg off the ground so that you have an extra stretch.
E) Reverse your position back to the starting position.
F) Repeat this exercise 10-15 times for each leg.

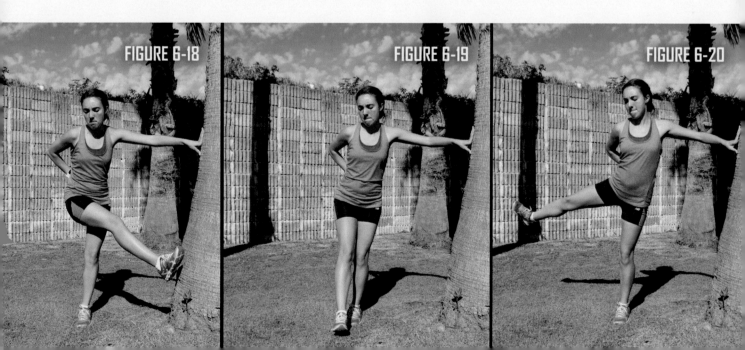

FIGURE 6-18   FIGURE 6-19   FIGURE 6-20

FORWARD LEG KICK
DRILL

The **Forward Leg Kick** drill improves the two key areas most often associated with loss of contact: hamstring and hip inflexibility. It does so while warming you up for race walking at the same time.

If there were two drills to perform before race walking, this and the **Side Leg Swing** drill should be at the top of the list.

BODY POSITION

Hold onto a pole or tree for balance.

STEPS

A) Extend your opposite arm and leg (Figure 6-23).
B) Swing the leg and hip under the body, while bringing the opposite arm back toward the body (Figure 6-22).
C) Drive the knee up as high as you can, while bringing your opposite arm back behind your body (Figure 6-21).
D) Reverse your arm and leg swing, extending back to your original position.

Repeat this exercise 10-15 times for each leg.

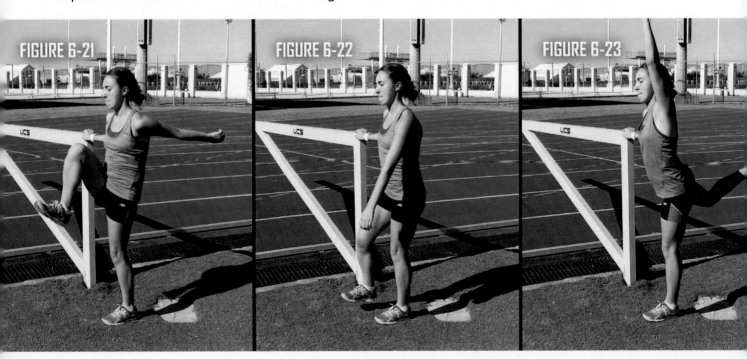

FIGURE 6-21   FIGURE 6-22   FIGURE 6-23

The following drills were introduced in previous chapters.

BEND DOWN HAMSTRING DRILL

We all need to stretch our hamstrings more. Since tight hamstrings make it difficult to maintain a straightened leg once the torso passes over it, a tight hamstring leads to pulling your rear foot off the ground prematurely, resulting in lifting.

This exercise is a great way to achieve a better range of motion from your hamstrings, while warming them up before a training walk.

See Chapter 5, page 48.

LONG STRIDES - LONG ARMS DRILL

There are many benefits to this drill. From a perspective of legality, a lack of forward hip rotation has the same effect as tight hamstrings; it leads to your rear foot coming off the ground prematurely. This is often due to tight hip flexors.

The beauty of this drill is that it increases the range of motion of the hips in a manner specific to race walking. Sometimes the lack of forward hip rotation in beginner walkers may be due to having difficulty understanding what hip rotation should feel like.

The **Long Strides – Long Arms** drill help beginning walkers exaggerate their hips forward with each stride. Finally, when the body is cold, this is a great way to get blood pumping to all extremities quickly.

See chapter 5, page 47.

EASY ON THE BACK
STRETCH

Walkers with really tight hamstrings or lower back problems may wish to start by using the *Easy on the Back Hamstring* stretch as a low-stress stretch after warming up.

BODY POSITION

Lie on the ground and stretch your one leg out.

STEPS

A) Lift the opposite leg, holding it as straight as you can (Figure 6-24); The more flexible you are, the closer to your torso you should be able to pull your leg.
B) Take care not to pull your other leg up from the ground.
C) Ideally, the leg you are stretching should be perpendicular to the ground; however, always stretch within your own limits.
D) You can use a rope or towel to assist getting a better stretch.
E) Hold the stretch for 20-30 seconds and repeat 2-3 times with each leg.

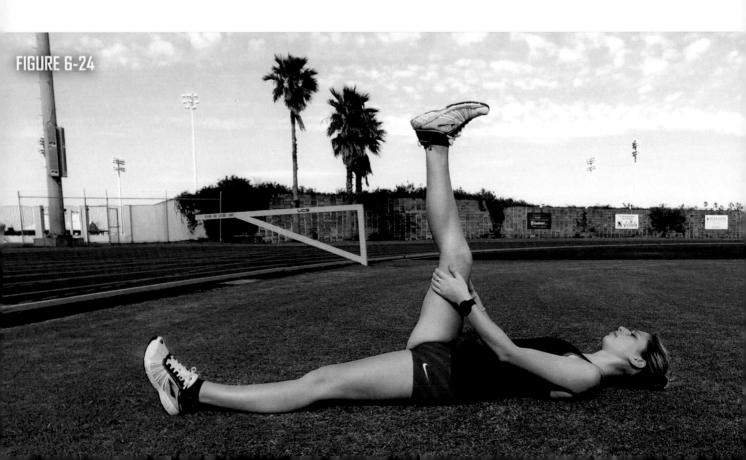

FIGURE 6-24

TOE TOUCHING HAMSTRING
STRETCH

Do you remember being asked to bend over and touch your toes in gym class? Good idea, bad execution. Bending over like that might cause stress to the lower back. Avoid problems by using the **Toe Touching Hamstring** stretch.

BODY POSITION

Instead of standing straight up, lean against a wall or pole.

STEPS

A) Keeping your buttocks against the pole, place your feet approximately six inches to one foot away.
B) Continue leaning against the wall while you bend down. Raise your toes and try to touch them (Figures 6-25 through 6-27).
C) Focus on preventing your legs from bending.
D) Keeping your feet away from the wall reduces the stress on your back and avoids straining the sciatic nerve, one of the largest nerves in your body.
E) Hold the stretch for 20-30 seconds and repeat 2-3 times.

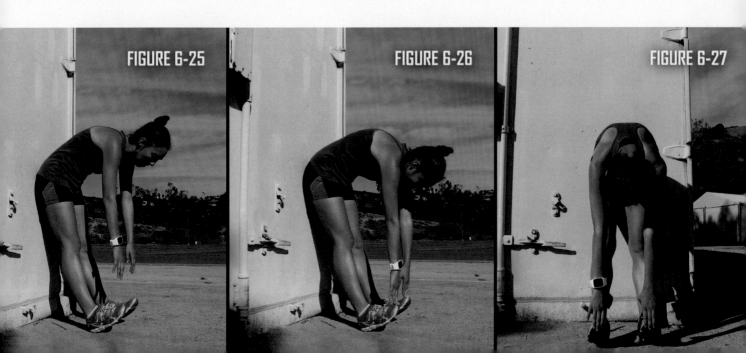

FIGURE 6-25   FIGURE 6-26   FIGURE 6-27

IMPROVED TOE TOUCHING HAMSTRING
STRETCH

Sometimes it's not convenient to lean against a wall or sit on the ground when you need to stretch your hamstrings. The **Improved Toe Touching Hamstring** stretch is almost identical to the **Toe Touching Hamstring** stretch, although it does not require a wall.

BODY POSITION

Stand straight up, but cross your feet.

STEPS

A) Keeping your buttocks your feet to remove the stress from your lower back, bend down and try to touch your toes; Focus on preventing your legs from bending.
B) Reach as far as you can without causing pain (Figures 6-28 & 6-29).
C) Hold the stretch for 20-30 seconds.
D) Cross your feet in the opposite manner and repeat steps A-C.
E) Note this is shown with a wall, but it is entirely optional.

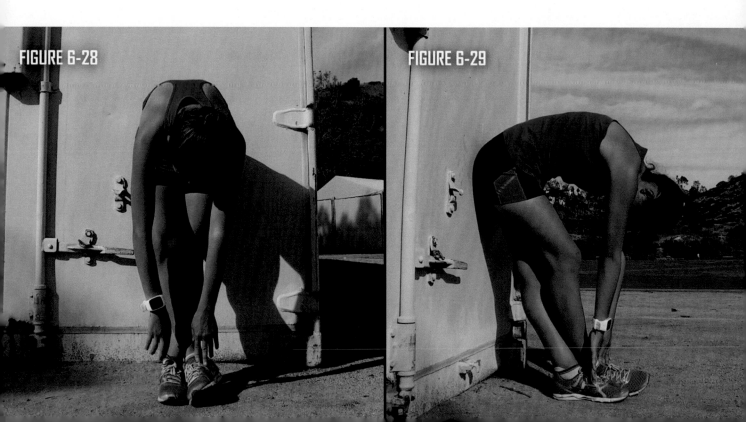

FIGURE 6-28   FIGURE 6-29

YOGA STYLE HAMSTRING STRETCH

Progressing through *Yoga Style Hamstring* stretch slowly stretches your neck, back, and hamstrings.

BODY POSITION

Begin in the same stance as with the *Toe Touching Hamstring* stretch then lower just your head, tucking your chin toward your chest (Figure 6-31).

STEPS

A) Slowly curl your upper body down and away from the wall (Figure 6-32).
B) Gradually allow your hands to drop to your sides; progress slowly lowering your hands toward your toes. Touch them if you can. Try to spend 20 to 30 seconds progressing to this point.
C) Finally, hang for another 10 to 20 seconds before reversing the process (Figure 6-35).
D) Reverse the stretch very gradually, concentrating on the sensation of your vertebrae stacking as you progress upwards.

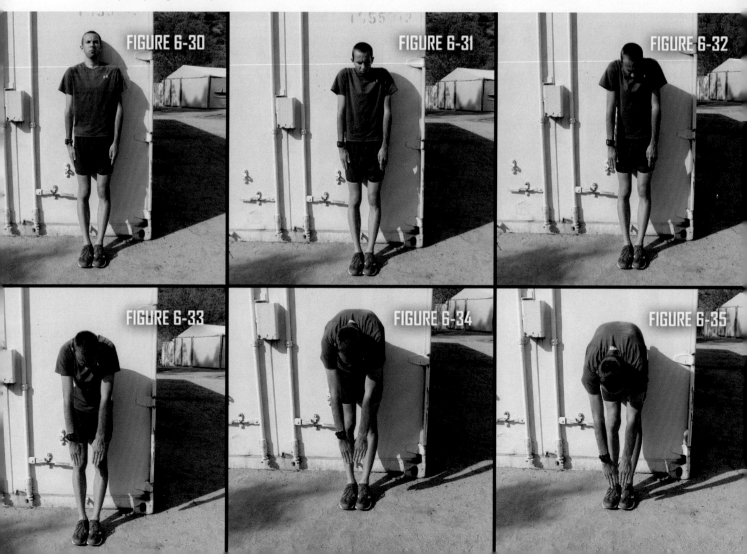

FIGURE 6-30   FIGURE 6-31   FIGURE 6-32

FIGURE 6-33   FIGURE 6-34   FIGURE 6-35

The following drills were introduced in previous chapters.

TRADITIONAL HAMSTRING STRETCH

The **Traditional Hamstring** stretch is an effective seated stretch of the hamstrings and an excellent post-training cool down. By isolating the hamstring muscle specifically, you minimize loss of contact issues. See chapter 5, page 64.

LEG UP HAMSTRING STRETCH

Sometimes getting down on the ground to stretch your hamstring isn't very convenient. Instead, try stretching your hamstrings standing up using the **Leg Up Hamstring** stretch. See chapter 5, page 65.

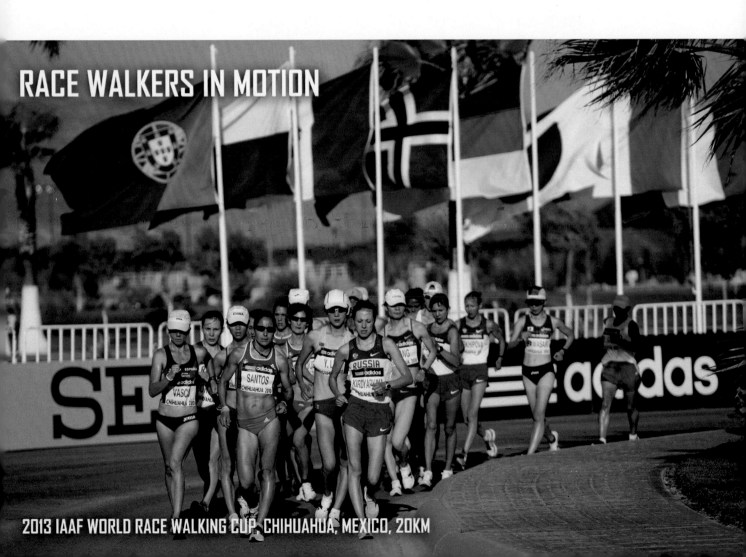

RACE WALKERS IN MOTION

2013 IAAF WORLD RACE WALKING CUP, CHIHUAHUA, MEXICO, 20KM

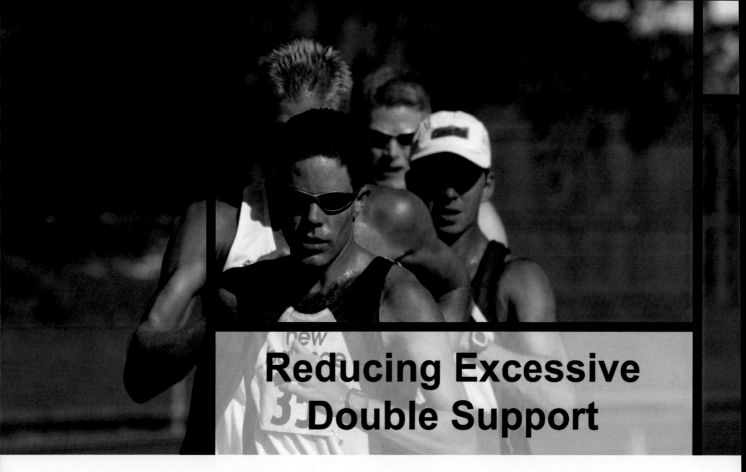

Reducing Excessive Double Support

Once you've mastered legal race walking technique there are many other tweaks required to reach efficient, ideal technique. Let's start by looking at a common issue with beginner walkers.

When race walkers first learn the technique, they do not usually exhibit the ideal timing of contacting the ground with the forward heel just as they roll off the toe of the back foot with the briefest of double-support contact phases.

Instead, a lack of strength, flexibility and perhaps a little too much weight around the belly lead to an excessively long double-support phase where both feet are on the ground at the same time.

Elite walkers, unless they have hit the wall, walk with no or a very minimal double-support phase. A smooth transition from the rear foot pushing off the ground to riding over the lead leg is a must. If both your front foot and rear foot are in contact with the ground for an extended duration, then while your rear foot is pushing off to propel you forward (Figure 7-1), its force is counterbalanced by the braking action of your front foot (Figure 7-2). This adds stress and can lead to injuries.

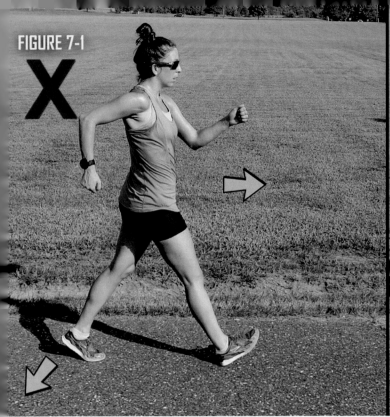

FIGURE 7-1

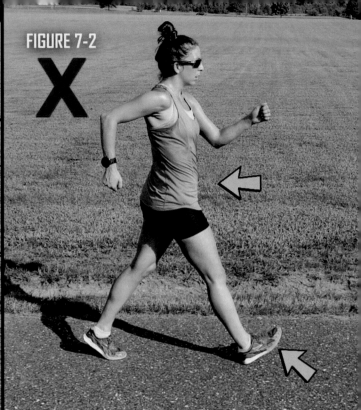

FIGURE 7-2

Focus and drills fix an excessive double-support phase.

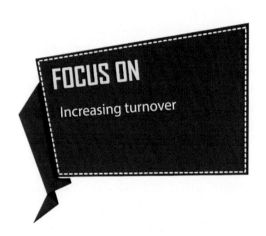

FOCUS ON
Increasing turnover

Focus on increasing the turnover rate of your feet. Pick your feet up and put them down at a faster rate to increase your cadence. Elite walkers walk at an average of approximately 200 steps per minute. A beginning walker averages closer to 150 steps per minute. With a little focus you can narrow the gap.

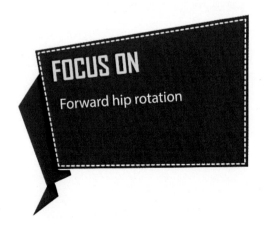

FOCUS ON
Forward hip rotation

We can't say enough times that it's all in the hips. Rotating your hips effectively lengthens your stride behind your body. One reason why people overstride is that they are trying to achieve a longer stride length. However, by reaching in front of the body with the leg you are not propelling your body forward. In actuality, you are slowing your progress. On the other hand, if your stride length increases due to good forward hip rotation, the increase in your stride is behind the body, where it can help to propel you forward.

Put a little oomph in your stride with a flick off your big toe. By pushing off your big toe, when your foot is behind the torso, you drive your body forward with more force. The additional force helps to reduce your double-support phase. However, be careful. If you push off prematurely, your body is pushed upward instead of forward.

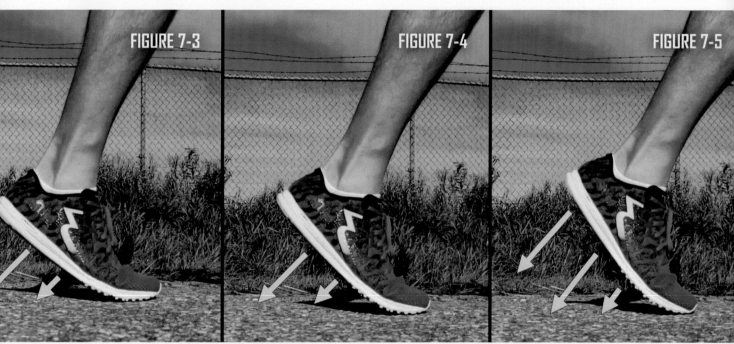

FIGURE 7-3   FIGURE 7-4   FIGURE 7-5

Training can improve your style if you lack leg speed or are overweight. Obviously, more training can lead to greater weight loss and therefore an improved style. If you lack leg speed, add a rhythm / economy workout once a week.

One of our favorites is Bohdan Bulakowski's workout of 100-, 200-, and 300-meter sets with 100 meters of walking easy in between. This is a great workout to get you on your toes with your legs moving quickly. See the book *Race Walk Faster by Training Smarter* for more detailed information about training.

QUICK STEPS DRILL

There are four variations of **Quick Step** drills that help to increase your speed, increase your turnover rate, and reduce overstriding. In addition, these drills allow you to practice getting your toes up. They also force you to straighten your knee as quickly as possible. Each variation follows the same basic steps.

BODY POSITION

Race walk with normal leg technique.

STEPS

A) Walk with very short strides of 12 inches or less.
B) Focus on turnover, forcing your feet to pick up and come down very quickly (Figures 7-6 through 7-8).
C) Focus on planting with your heel, landing with your toe up, and rolling through smoothly.
D) Focus on quieting your shoulders and torso.

The first two versions of **Quick Steps** are to place your **Hands Behind the Back** (Figure 7-9) or to place your **Hands Behind Your Head** (Figure 7-10). This causes the hips to be forced to move without the aid of the arms pumping forward and back, thus also helping you develop forward hip rotation.

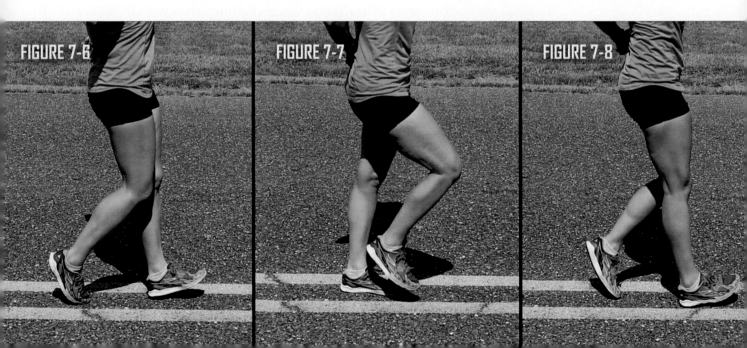

FIGURE 7-6

FIGURE 7-7

FIGURE 7-8

You can also try the **Superman** variation (Figure 7-11) where you place your hands out in front of your body and keep your head held as steady as possible. Excessive movement of the head could cause judges to think that you are lifting. Therefore, this is good practice not only for our feet, but also for our head.

A final variation of **Quick Steps** is the **Airplane** (Figure 7-12) where you place your hands out to your sides. This helps with turnover and forward hip rotation.

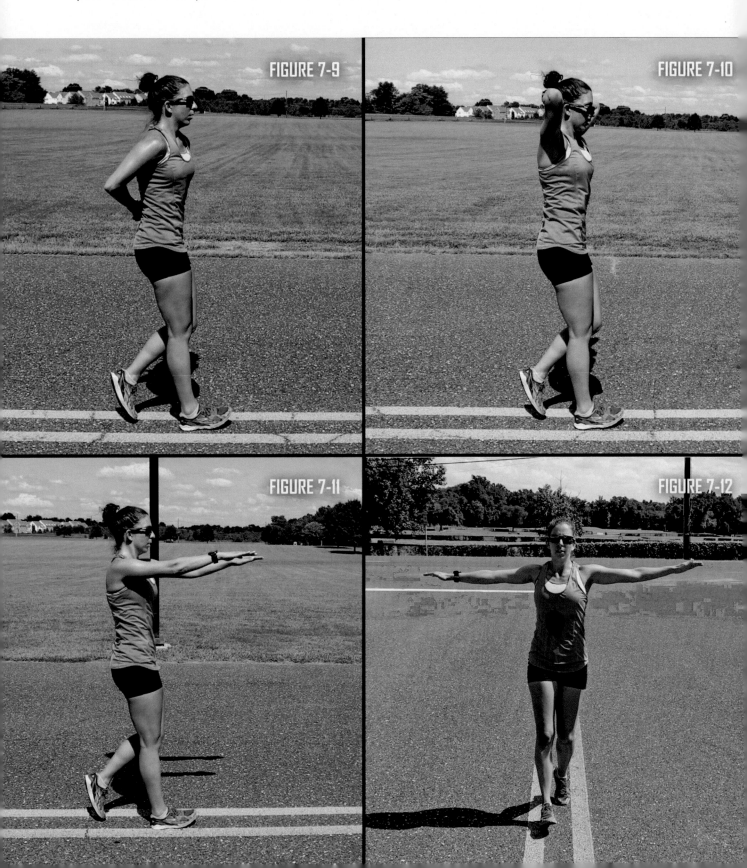

FIGURE 7-9   FIGURE 7-10   FIGURE 7-11   FIGURE 7-12

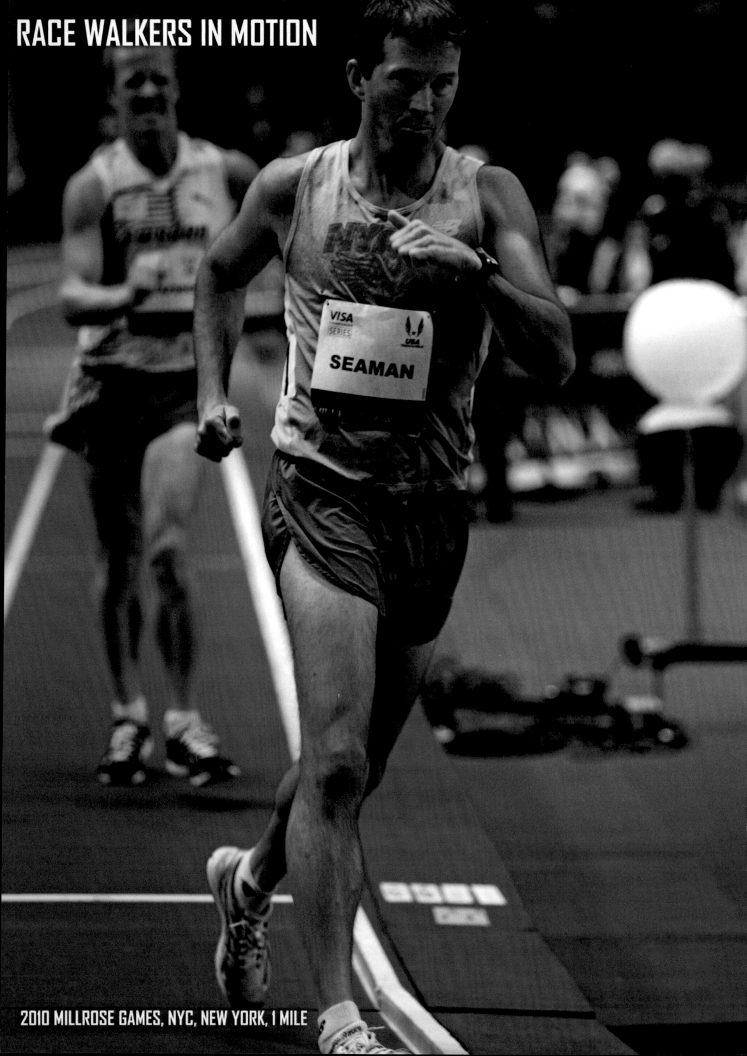

2010 MILLROSE GAMES, NYC, NEW YORK, 1 MILE

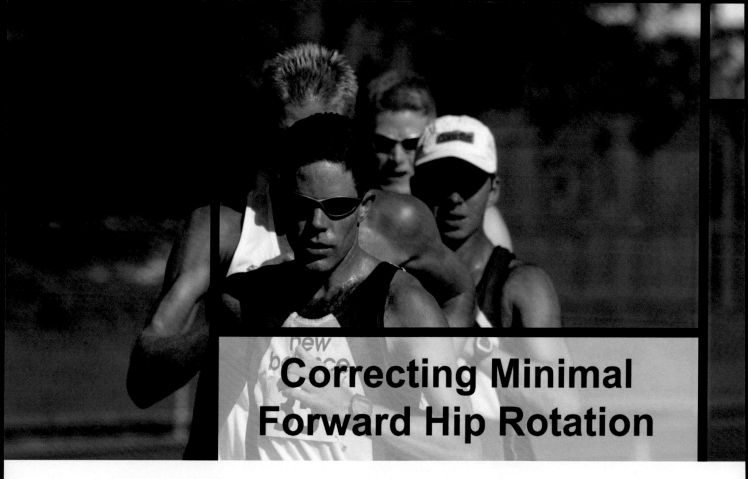

Correcting Minimal Forward Hip Rotation

Hips are the primary motor driving your body forward. Therefore, race walking can be incredibly frustrating to beginning walkers who cannot seem to get the feel of proper hip motion. Saying "use your hips more" just falls upon deaf ears. Walkers with minimal hip motion need drills and exercises to help them learn. Other race walkers may have hip motion, but in all the wrong directions.

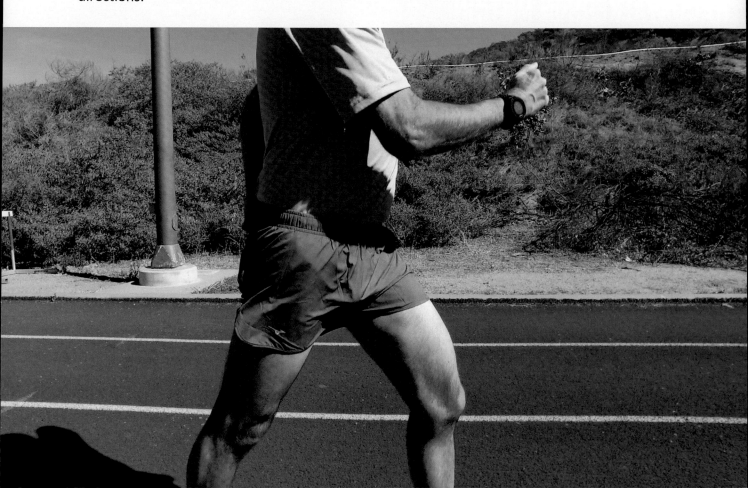

We will demonstrate how to correct both problems. If you are having difficulty feeling the proper motion of the hips, try two drills that help you feel forward hip rotation.

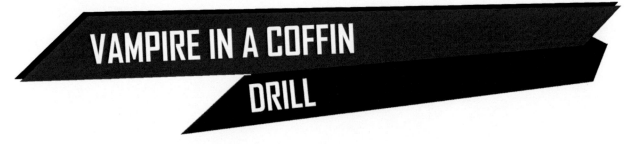

Review the drill where we engage our hips by acting like a vampire in Chapter 4, Page 30.

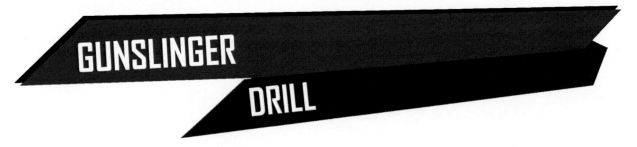

Review the drill / analogy where we pretend to be a gunslinger in the old west to mimic forward hip rotation in Chapter 4, Page 31.

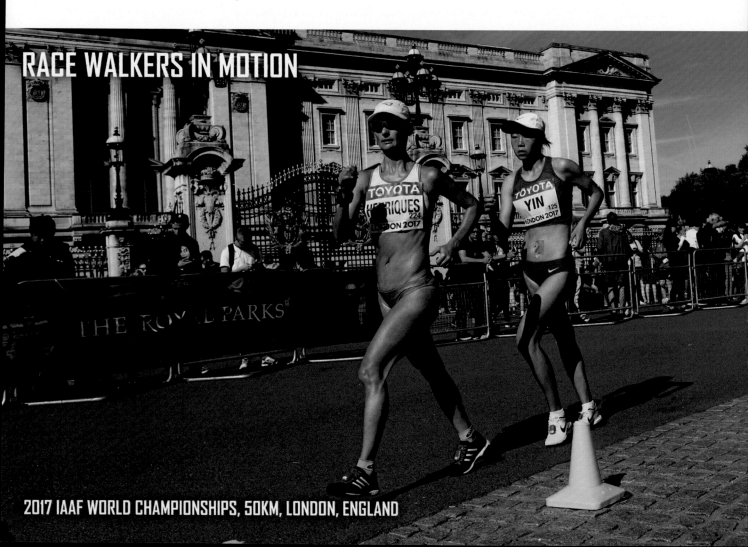

RACE WALKERS IN MOTION

2017 IAAF WORLD CHAMPIONSHIPS, 50KM, LONDON, ENGLAND

FUNKY HIP DRILL
DRILL

The **Funky Hip Drill** stretches the hip in a manner consistent with race walking technique. This improves the fluidity of the hip motion.

BODY POSITION

Stand with both feet on the ground as in double-support phase of race walking.

STEPS

A) With your right leg forward and your arms behind your back, raise the toes of your right foot, like when you plant your heel in race walking.
B) Shift your weight to that leg, making sure that your leg is straightened.
C) Push your right hip to the outside, so that your right IT band (Iliotibial band, facia around tissue reaching from your hip down to your knee); This stretches from where it connects to the knee up to where it connects in the hip (Figure 8-1).
D) Reverse the steps for your other leg (Figure 8-2).
E) Walk forward repeating the drill for 30 meters.

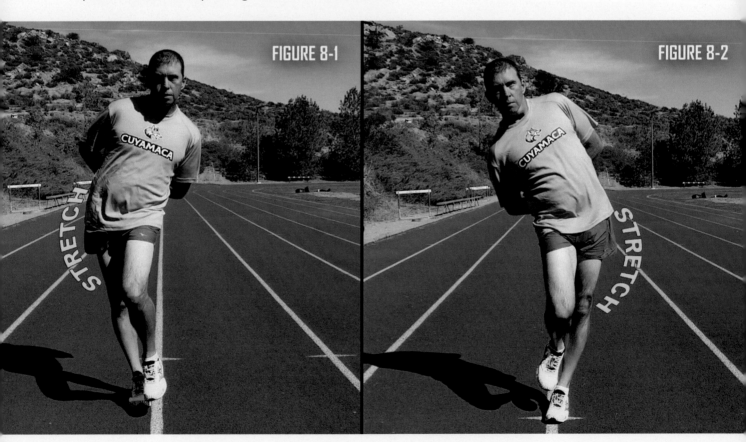

FIGURE 8-1   FIGURE 8-2

ARM SWINGS WITH ELASTIC BANDS DRILL

There is nothing better than performing a drill with the same motion as race walking. The single best arm exercise for race walking is to practice the motion of the race walker's arm swings with elastic bands so that you use your hips properly. The enhanced arm swing forces a greater forward rotation of the hips. Also, if performed in front of a mirror, this exercise can help you develop proper arm motion.

BODY POSITION

Wrap an elastic band around a pole (or anything stable) and place each end in your hands.

STEPS

A) Swing the hands forward and backward through the full range of motion traveled while race walking.
B) Counter your arm swing by pushing your opposite hip forward (Figures 8-3 & 8-4).
C) Remember to keep those shoulders relaxed!
D) Repeat this exercise for 2 to 10 minutes.

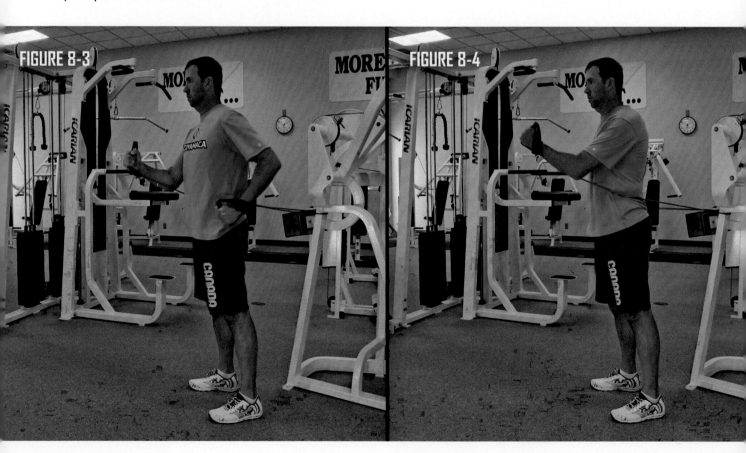

FIGURE 8-3   FIGURE 8-4

TIM'S STRETCH

Since Tim doesn't remember where he learned this hip flexor stretch or what it was called, he now claims it by his own name. Good hip flexor range of motion is a key to good forward hip rotation.

BODY POSITION

Sit on the floor with your weight resting on a bent right leg.

STEPS

A) Place your left leg behind the body and bend it at the knee to approximately 90 degrees.
B) Use your right elbow to support your upper body weight.
C) Raise your left elbow above the head and arch your back, while also slightly pushing your left hip forward (Figure 8-5). This gives a nice long line to follow from the left hip to the left elbow, allowing for a great stretch from the left hip flexor all the way up to the left triceps.
D) Repeat with your right side of your body.

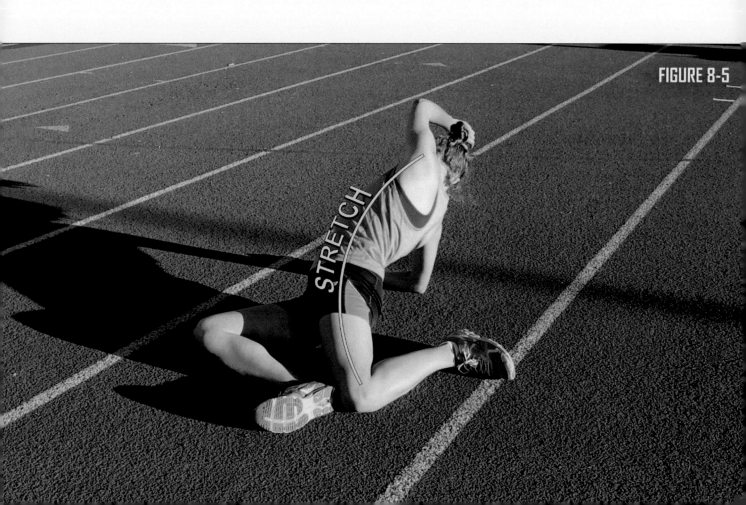

FIGURE 8-5

STRETCH

SIDE
STRETCH

The *Side* stretch provides a good stretch from where the IT band connects to the knee all the way up to the elbow. Stretching this area facilitates good forward hip rotation.

BODY POSITION

Stand with both feet together.

STEPS

A) Grab your right elbow with your left hand.
B) Bend your left knee while keeping the right knee straight.
C) Hold for 20-30 seconds (Figure 8-6).
D) Return to the vertical position.
E) Repeat 2-3 times on one side, then switch and repeat on the other side.

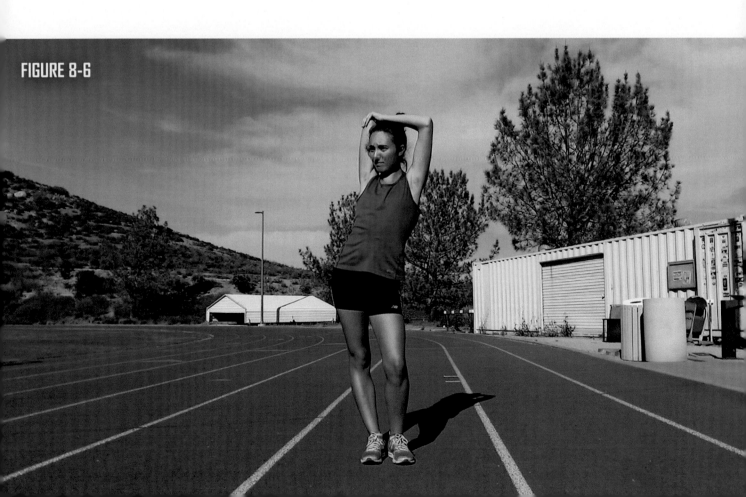

FIGURE 8-6

ADVANCED SIDE
STRETCH

The **Advanced Side** Stretch drill is another version of the **Side** stretch drill to improve stretching the side and IT band.

BODY POSITION

Stand with your legs crossed over each other, but your feet close together.

STEPS

A) Grab your left elbow with your right hand.
B) Slightly bend your right knee while keeping the left knee straight.
C) Hold for 20-30 seconds (Figure 8-7).
D) Return to the vertical position.
E) Repeat 2-3 times on one side, then switch and repeat on the other side.

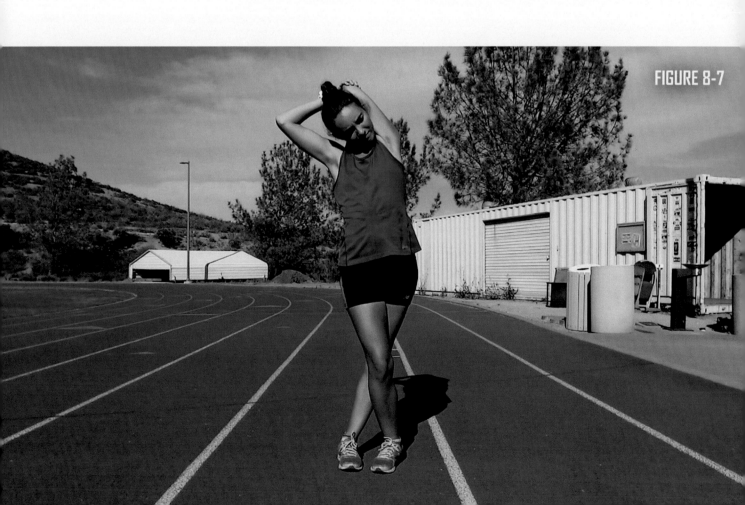

FIGURE 8-7

IT BAND
STRETCH

The **IT Band** stretch is yet another activity to loosen up the IT band. It's important to find a stretch that works for you as a tight IT band not only restricts forward hip rotation, but can lead to knee injuries as well.

BODY POSITION

Stand with one leg crossed in front of the other.

STEPS

A) Place your hands together and bend to your side.
B) Lean in the opposite direction of your hands and push the hip out slightly.
C) Hold for 20-30 seconds and repeat 2-3 times on each side (Figures 8-8 & 8-9).

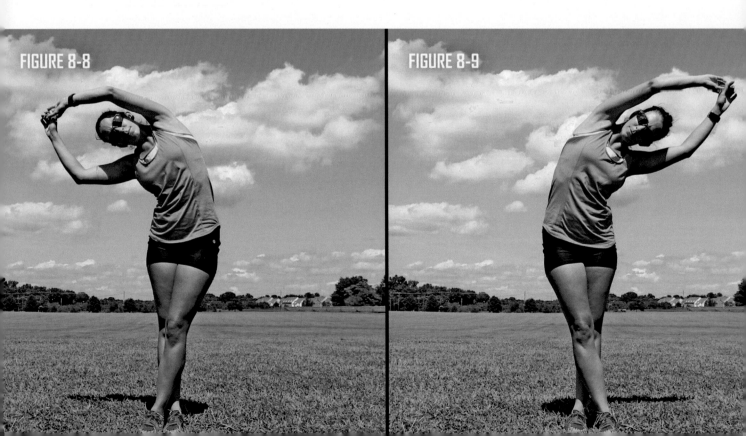

FIGURE 8-8

FIGURE 8-9

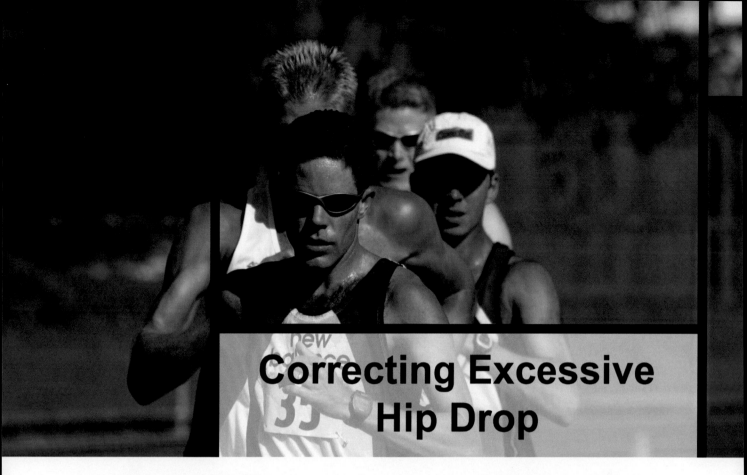

Correcting Excessive Hip Drop

Excessive hip drop is a tricky issue for some race walkers. Part of the problem could be a misconception as to how the hip moves. While the hip has to move up and down, many race walkers falsely assume that it should be a more excessive vertical movement. For those walkers, correcting the problem is simply a matter of relearning the proper motion.

Other walkers, however, suffer from a lack of, or imbalance of strength and flexibility in the hips and core which causes the excessive hip drop. Often, when the hip drops, it also sways outward. While these two motions could occur independently, they are usually observed together. The hip sway compensates for the drop in center of gravity that is caused by the hip drop. Here are a series of exercises and stretches to help correct excessive hip drop and sway.

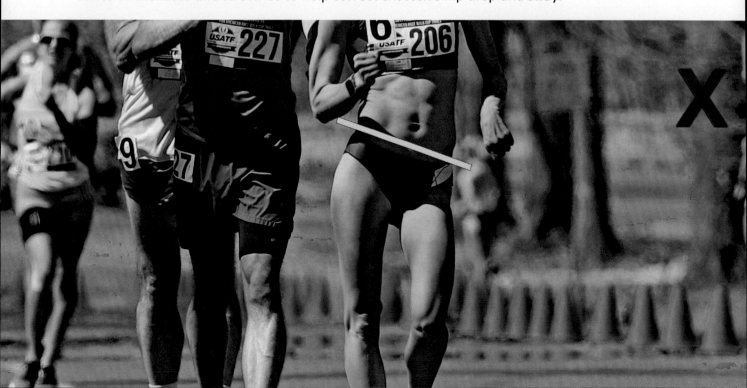

STRAIGHT LINE WALKING DRILL

A side effect of rotating your hips forward is that your feet land in a straight line. Therefore, when you perform the **Straight Line Walking** drill by literally race walking along a straight line, your tendency to sway outward with your hip is reduced.

BODY POSITION

This drill is performed while race walking.

STEPS

A) Race walk along a straight line, such as a lane divider of a track (Figures 9-1 & 9-2).

B) As you walk, focus on your hips, reaching forward as the advancing leg swings forward.

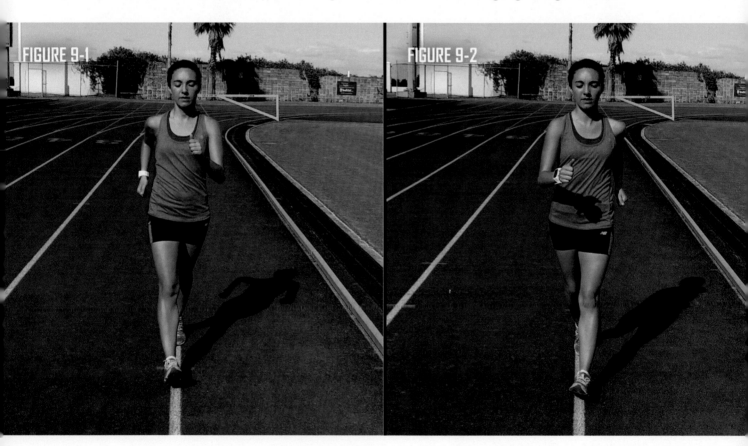

FIGURE 9-1

FIGURE 9-2

LONG STRIDES - LONG ARMS
DRILL

If you are swaying to the side instead of driving your hip forward, resynchronize your hips by doing the **Long Strides – Long Arms** drill.

See chapter 5, page 47 for steps to complete this drill.

CLAM SHELL
EXERCISE

The *Clam Shell Exercise* strengthens your hip abductors to prevent your hip from dropping excessively.

BODY POSITION

Lie on your side.

STEPS

A) Position your legs so that they are in a clam shell position.
B) Raise and lower the upper leg, maintaining the V (Figures 9-3 & 9-4).
C) Repeat 2-3 sets of 20 reps with the same leg.
D) Repeat with the other leg.

For an added effort, place a light weight on the upper leg or use resistance bands between the thighs.

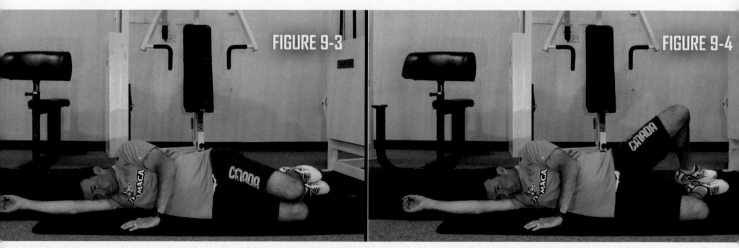

FIGURE 9-3   FIGURE 9-4

BRIDGE WITH BALL
EXERCISE

The **Bridge with Ball** exercise strengthens the lower back muscles and hamstrings. This is a complementary exercise that helps but is not specific to one hip rotation problem.

BODY POSITION

Lie on your back.

STEPS

A) Place your feet on an exercise ball.
B) Place your hands at your side.
C) While exhaling, raise your butt from the floor and hold for 2 to 3 seconds (Figure 9-5).
D) While inhaling, lower your butt back to the floor.
E) Repeat up to 20 times; do 2 sets.

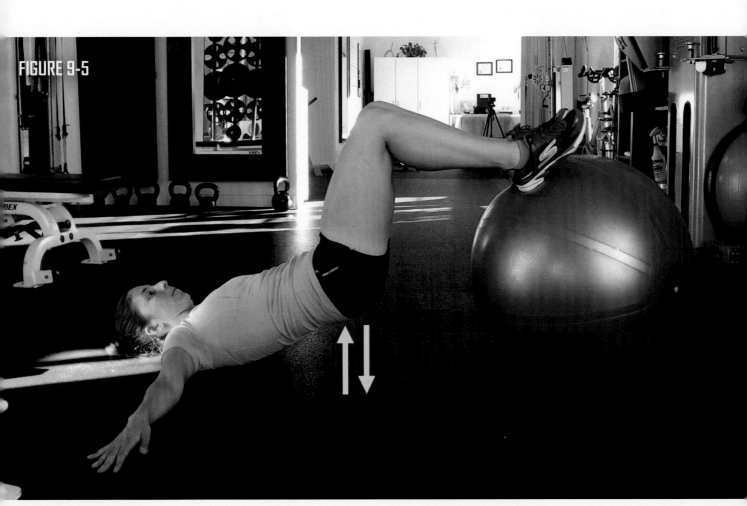

FIGURE 9-5

ELASTIC BAND - LEG STRAP
EXERCISE

The **Elastic Band Leg Strap** *Exercise* strengthens your hip abductors to help in preventing your hip from dropping excessively.

BODY POSITION

Place an elastic band around your lower legs and stand in a partial squat position with your legs a shoulder's width apart.

STEPS

A) Slowly walk from side to side.

B) Move a few side steps in one direction, then a few steps back in the original direction (Figures 9-6 & 9-7).

C) Take caution to make sure that each foot moves the same distance on each step.

D) Repeat 10 to 20 times.

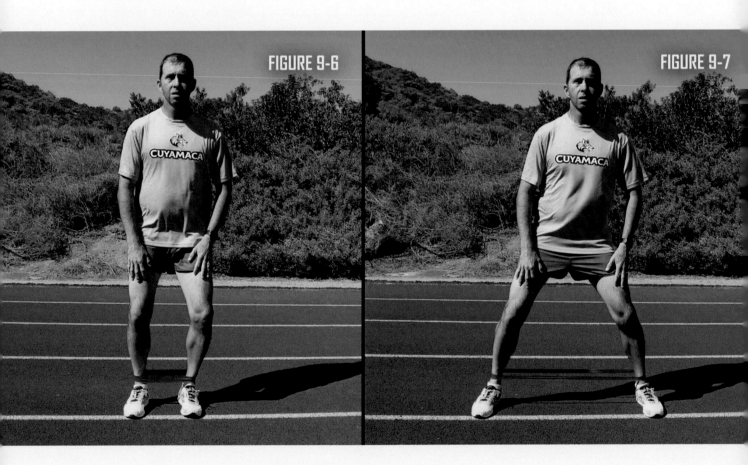

FIGURE 9-6   FIGURE 9-7

SIDE STRAIGHT LEG RAISE
EXERCISE

For those with excessive hip drop, the **Side Straight Leg Raise** exercise strengthens the hip abductors without the need to go to the gym. Weak hip abductors are one reason the hip may drop excessively in race walking.

This exercise can be done with or without a light ankle weight. Start without weight and gradually add light weights, building up to but never exceeding 10 percent of your body weight.

BODY POSITION

Lay on your side with both legs extended. Your lower leg may be slightly bent for balance, while your top leg should be fully extended. Additionally, your lower arm is extended, and your upper arm is used for support.

STEPS

A) Slowly raise the top leg, while keeping it straight, to about 45 degrees; hold it there for a second, and then gradually lower it (Figure 9-8).
B) Repeat this exercise 20 times with one leg, then switch and repeat with the other leg.

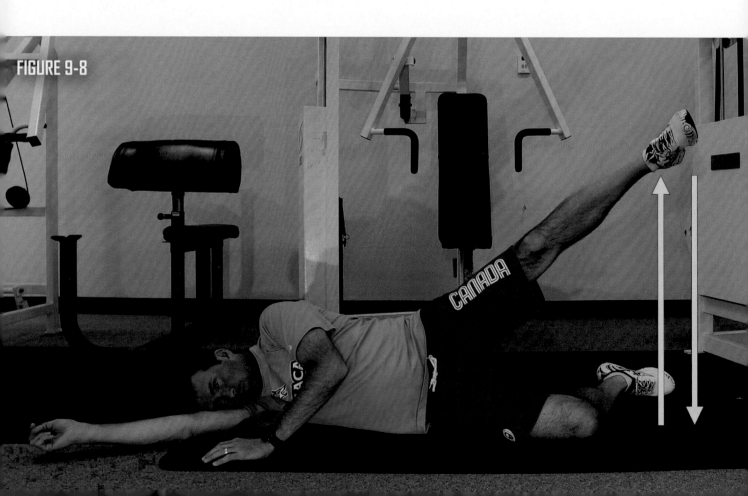

FIGURE 9-8

LOWER SIDE STRAIGHT LEG RAISE
EXERCISE

For those with excessive hip drop, the **Lower Side Straight Leg Raise** exercise strengthens the hip adductors without the need to go to the gym. Weak hip adductors are one reason the hip may drop excessively in race walking.

This exercise can be done with or without a light ankle weight. Start without weight and gradually add light weights, building up to but never exceeding 5 percent of your body weight.

BODY POSITION

Lay on your side with the lower leg extended out straight and the upper leg bent in a triangular position. Additionally, your lower arm is extended, and your upper arm is used for support.

STEPS

A) Slowly raise the lower leg, while keeping it straight, to about 15 degrees; hold it there for a second, and then gradually lower it (Figure 9-9).
B) Repeat this exercise 20 times with one leg, then switch and repeat with the other leg.

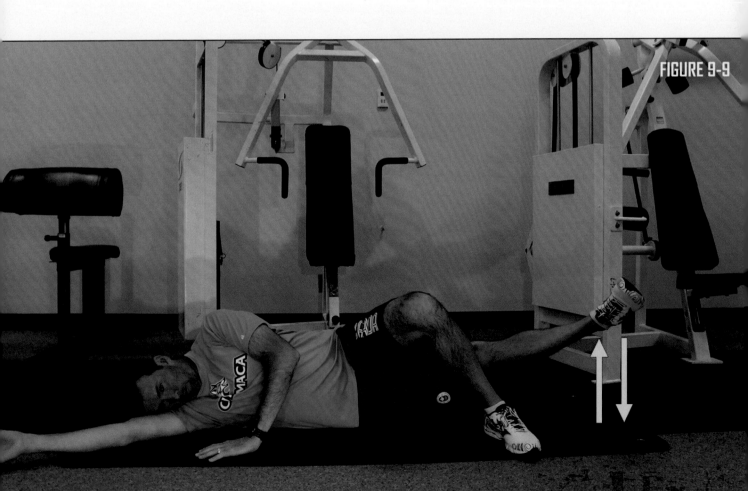

FIGURE 9-9

HIP FLEXOR - LUNGE FORWARD
STRETCH

The **Hip Flexor – Lunge Forward** stretch is great for working on tight hip flexors which inhibit proper forward hip rotation.

BODY POSITION

Place your right knee on the ground with your right foot extended behind you. Place your left foot on the ground in front of you, making sure the left knee stays behind the ankle

STEPS

A) With a straight back, lunge forward and feel the stretch in your right hip flexor (Figures 9-10 & 9-11).
B) Hold for 20-30 seconds.
C) Repeat 2-3 times on each side.
D) For an advanced stretch, raise both your hands while keeping your back in a vertical position (Figure 9-12).

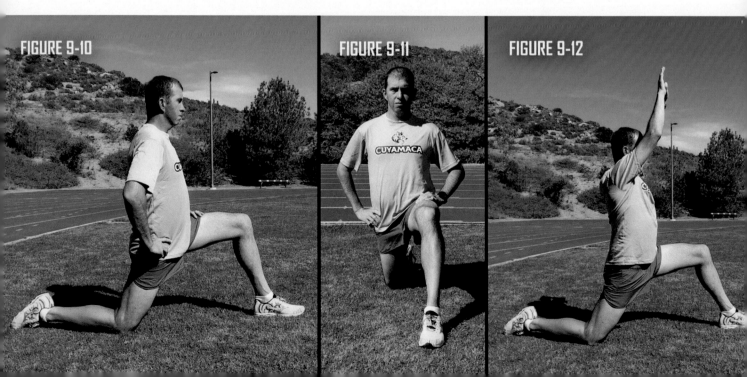

FIGURE 9-10   FIGURE 9-11   FIGURE 9-12

PIRIFORMIS STRETCH

The **_Piriformis_** stretch is great for stretching the muscle located within the glutes. Due to the excess hip rotation of a race walker's stride, this muscle tends to tighten, which can lead to an injury known as piriformis syndrome.

BODY POSITION

Lay on back.

STEPS

A) Place your right foot on your left knee.
B) Lift your left knee up so that your thigh is perpendicular with the ground.
C) Grab your leg under the knee and pull the leg toward you (Figure 9-13).
D) Hold for 20-30 seconds.
E) Repeat 2-3 times with each leg.

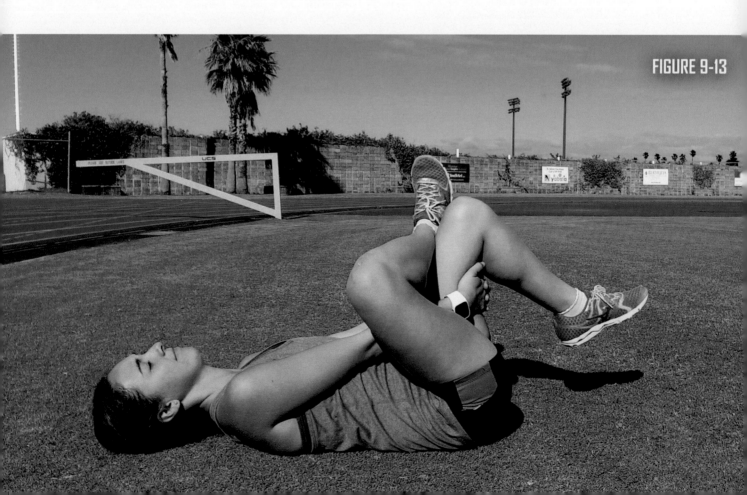

FIGURE 9-13

ADVANCED HIP FLEXOR STRETCH

Tight hip flexors inhibit proper forward hip rotation.

BODY POSITION

Kneel on the ground, preferably soft ground.

STEPS

A) Place your left leg in front of the body while bending at the knee.
B) Lower your torso, using your hands for support.
C) Slide the right leg back and lower your torso all the way down so that your forearms are supporting your body weight.
D) Feel the stretch across your right hip flexor and left piriformis.
E) Hold for 20-30 seconds.
F) Repeat 2-3 times for each side.

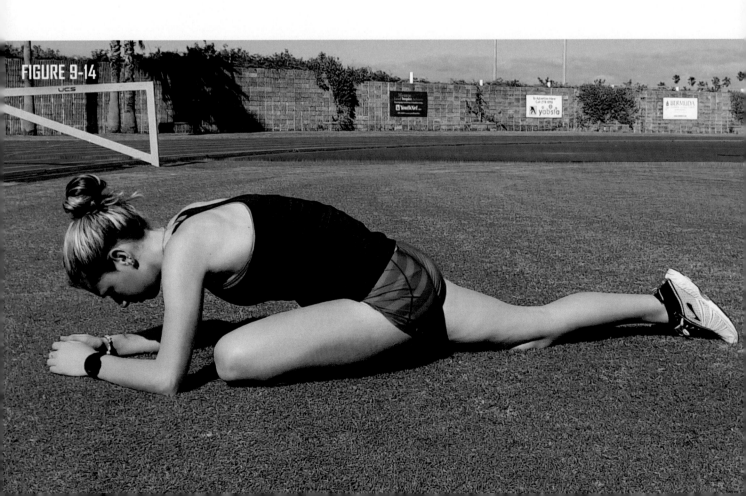

FIGURE 9-14

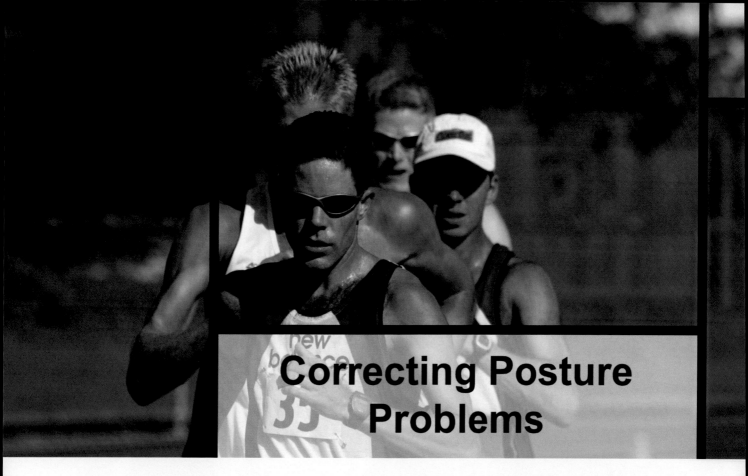

Correcting Posture Problems

Stand up straight! How many times have you heard that? It sounds easy, but it isn't always easy to accomplish. In ideal race walking posture, the torso is in the vertical position (Figure 10-2). Some race walkers never achieve this, while others develop problems when they become tired late in races. In general, posture problems fall into two main categories: leaning forward (Figure 10-1) and leaning backward (Figure 10-3).

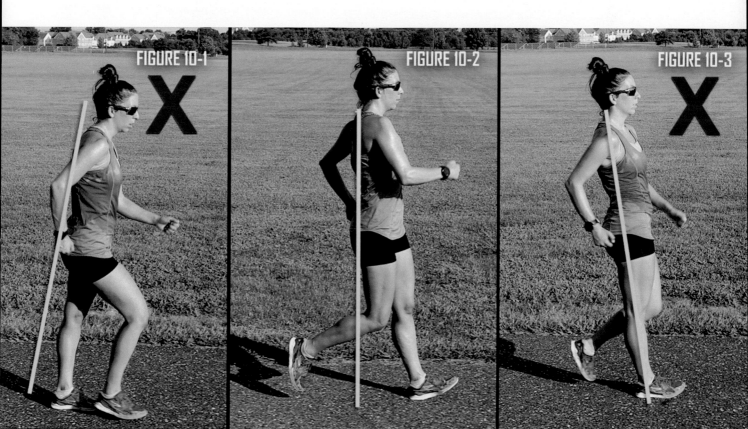

FIGURE 10-1 X

FIGURE 10-2

FIGURE 10-3 X

Good posture (Figure 10-5) also helps more of the stride to be behind the body instead of in front of the body. In contrast, leaning forward (Figure 10-4) or backward (Figure 10-6) restricts hip rotation and limits the stride behind the body. Many race walkers are not aware of the problems with their posture. With the availability of video cameras and high speed still photography, have someone take a video or series of photos of you race walking. Either stop on a frame or grab a still when your supporting leg is beneath your body. Draw a vertical line and compare it to your body position.

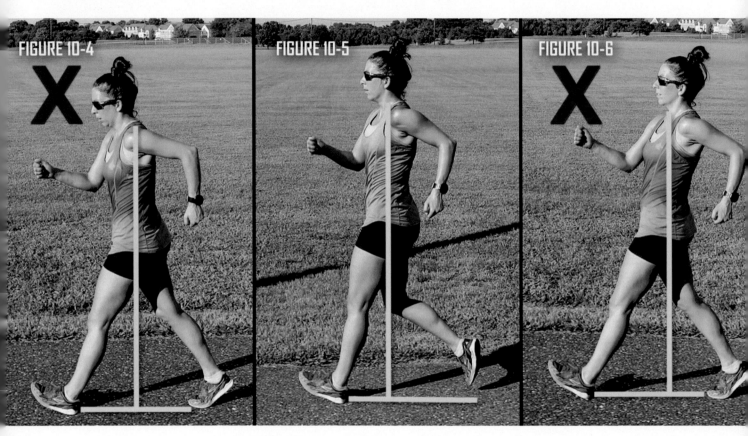

If you have an issue, here are some simple steps to help correct it.

Correcting Leaning Forward

Forward lean is very undesirable in race walking. It can be caused for many reasons, including poor coaching. The main physical causes are tight abdominal muscles, overdeveloped or tight pectoral muscles, weak lats (the biggest back muscle group), and/or a weak lower back. While focus alone won't correct all of your posture issues, it's a good place to start.

Your posture often follows your head position. If you drop your head (Figure 10-7), your posture is sure to follow, and you will slouch forward. When you race walk, focus on keeping your head up (Figure 10-8). Pay attention to your chin as well. Keeping it up helps to bring your posture upright as well as allowing your airway to stay open, letting your body get maximum oxygen when the going gets tough.

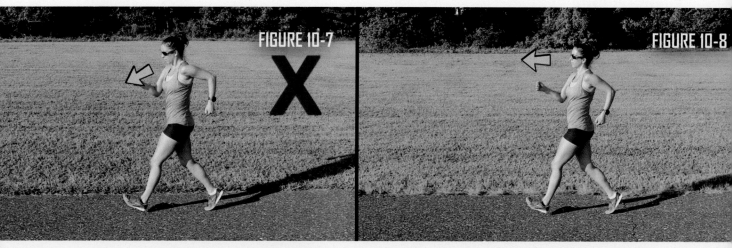
FIGURE 10-7   FIGURE 10-8

One challenge to correcting posture is that your posture issues may not be related to race walking. Your posture may be incorrect in your pedestrian style walk as well. If so, then you are correcting decades of bad habits and imbalance. One of the first steps is for you to feel what it feels like to actually walk in the vertical position.

If you have someone who can help you, have them place your body in the vertical position. If you previously leaned forward, you might feel like you are falling backward. Likewise, if you are leaning backwards, you might feel like you are falling forward. If you are alone or want more practice, you could also do this using a treadmill and mirror. Make a vertical line on the mirror to show where your body should be when you are walking on the treadmill. Focus on walking (positioning the mirror to the side of the treadmill) while keeping your body even with the line.

Next, we need to strengthen and improve the flexibility of the muscles causing you to lean forward. Do the following exercise three times per week.

ALTERNATE ARM AND LEG EXERCISE

This **Alternate Arm and Leg** exercise doesn't require a gym or even weights. It strengthens the lower back muscles as well as the glutes, hamstrings, and to some degree the shoulders and thus helps to correct forward lean.

BODY POSITION

Lying on your stomach, hold your arms and legs straight out.

STEPS

A) While exhaling, raise one arm and the opposite leg from the floor; Be sure to keep them mostly straight and inhale as you lower your limbs (Figure 10-9).
B) Exhale while raising the opposite arm and leg, keeping them mostly straight (Figure 10-10). Inhale as you lower them.
C) Repeat, 2 sets of 10.

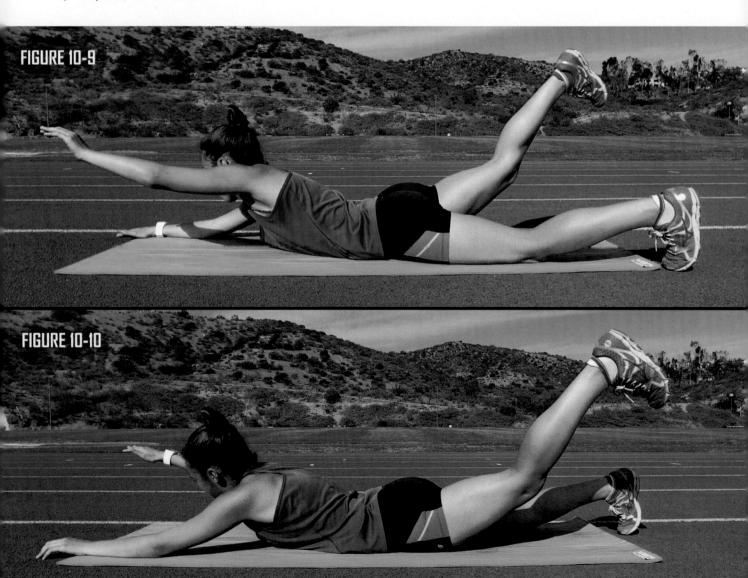

FIGURE 10-9

FIGURE 10-10

SUPERMAN EXERCISE

This exercise is a variation of the **Alternate Arm and Leg** exercise that also strengthens the lower back muscles as well as the glutes, hamstrings, and to some degree the shoulders.

BODY POSITION

Lying on your stomach, hold your arms and legs straight out (Figure 10-11).

STEPS

A) Simultaneously, exhale and raise your arms and legs off the floor (Figure 10-12); Be sure to keep them straight.
B) Hold for 3 seconds.
C) Inhale as you lower your arms and legs.
D) Repeat 15 times.

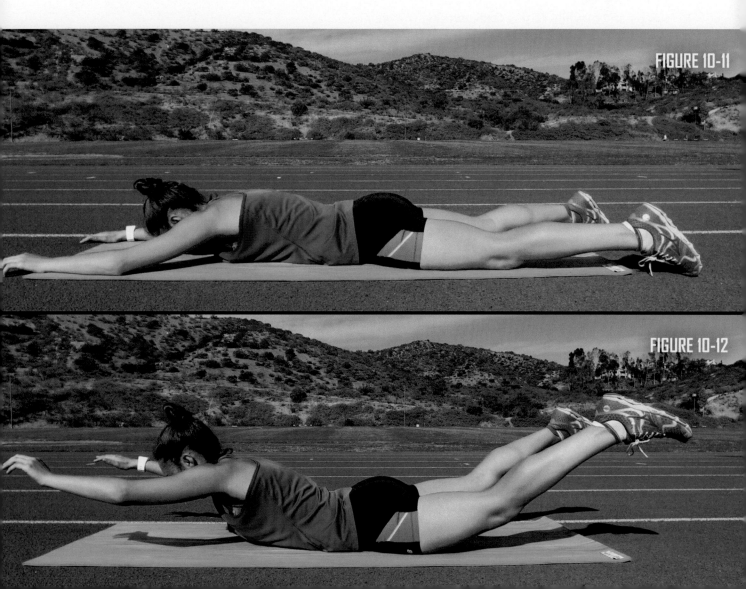

FIGURE 10-11

FIGURE 10-12

LAT PULLDOWN EXERCISE

This exercise helps to correct leaning forward because if your lats aren't strong enough, your torso will be pulled forward by your abdominal muscles. This is especially true for people who have done a lot of abdominal work while neglecting their back.

BODY POSITION

Sit in front of a lat machine.

STEPS

A) Grab the bar with your palms facing away from you, and place your hands at end of the bar.
B) While exhaling, pull the bar down in front of your body.
C) Lower the bar all the way down to past your chest (Figure 10-13).
D) Slowly, return the bar back to the top, stopping just before your arms completely straighten (Figure 10-14).
E) Keep control while raising and lowering the weight.
F) Don't let the bar swing back excessively as you return to a starting position.
G) Perform 10 repetitions for 3 sets.

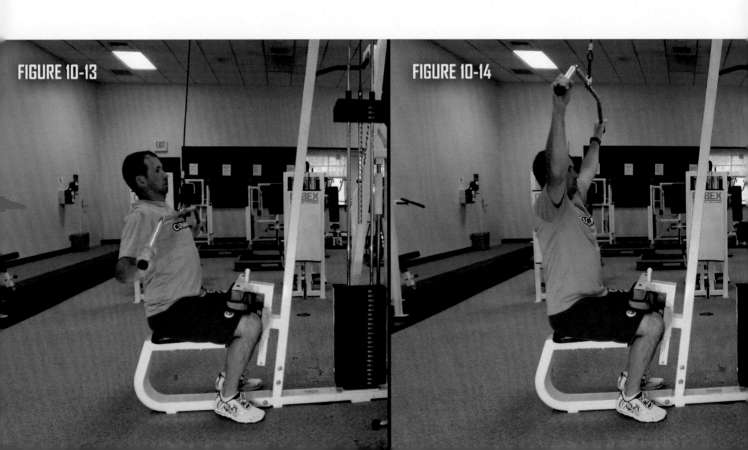

FIGURE 10-13

FIGURE 10-14

ROWING MACHINE
EXERCISE

If you already have strong pectoral muscles, the muscles located in your chest, a rowing machine balances by strengthening your rhomboids, which are located in your upper outer back, between your shoulder blades and your spine. Strengthening your rhomboids pulls you upright so that you don't lean forward.

BODY POSITION

Sit on the seat of a rowing machine.

STEPS

A) Grab the handles of the machine with straightened arms (Figure 10-15).
B) Pull back on the cable(s), keeping your back straight (Figure 10-16).
C) Inhale while you lower the weight by straightening your arms.
D) Repeat 20 times for 3 sets.

TAKE CARE!!!

Use the shoulders and shoulder blades to bring the cable backward. Do not over utilize your arm muscles.

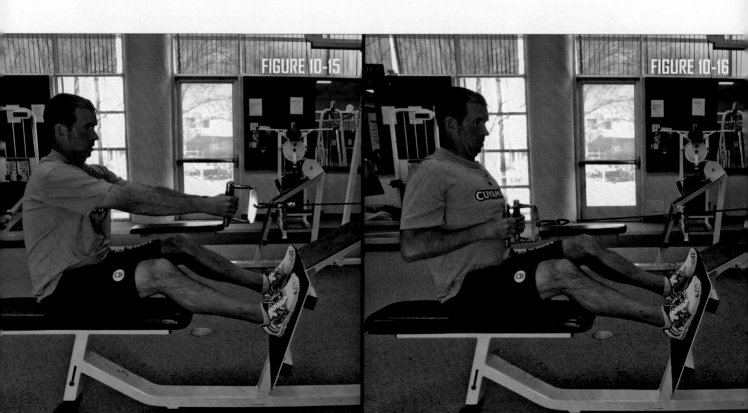

FIGURE 10-15

FIGURE 10-16

BACK EXTENSION
EXERCISE

For those with a healthy back, a back extension machine strengthens the lower back to hold you in a good upright posture and helps to correct leaning forward.

STEPS

Since there are many different types of back extension machines, follow the instructions at your local gym. Please do not try this exercise if you have back problems.

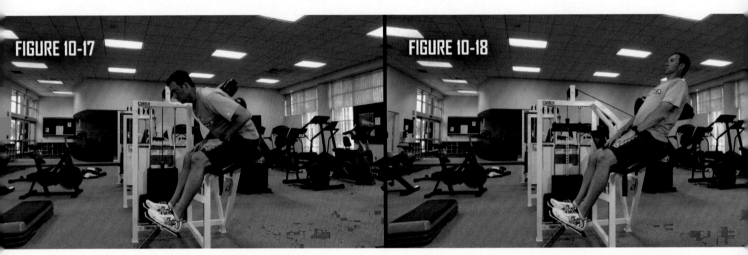

FIGURE 10-17 FIGURE 10-18

BRIDGE WITH BALL
EXERCISE

The *Bridge with Ball* exercise introduced in chapter 9, page 100 is a great way to strengthen and pull you posture backward into a vertical position.

PEC
STRETCH

Tight pectoral muscles pull your shoulders into a forward, rounded position, thus causing you to lean forward as you race walk. The **Pec** stretch loosens them.

BODY POSITION

Stand in a doorway.

STEPS

A) Place one arm against the doorway, holding your arm at an 80-degree angle with the side of your body.
B) Lean forward, maintaining a vertical body alignment, until you feel the stretch across your pecs (Figure 10-19).
C) Hold for 30 seconds.
D) If you don't feel the stretch, bend your arm at your elbow at a 90-degree angle.
E) Repeat five times on each side.

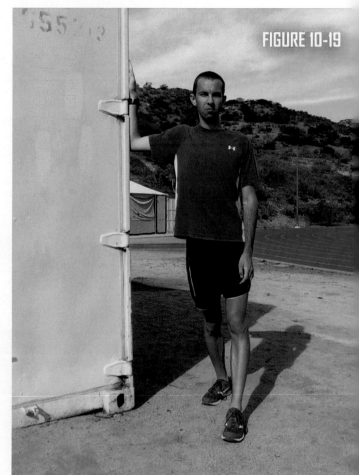

FIGURE 10-19

COBRA
STRETCH

This stretch corrects leaning forward if your abdominals are tight. It stretches them into extension.

BODY POSITION

Lie face down, extending your legs behind you with your feet together.

STEPS

A) Place your hands on the side of your body, even with your shoulders (Figure 10-20).
B) Keeping your legs on the floor and feet flat, push your body up while exhaling (Figure 10-21).
C) Hold for five seconds.
D) Lower your body down while inhaling.
E) Repeat ten times.

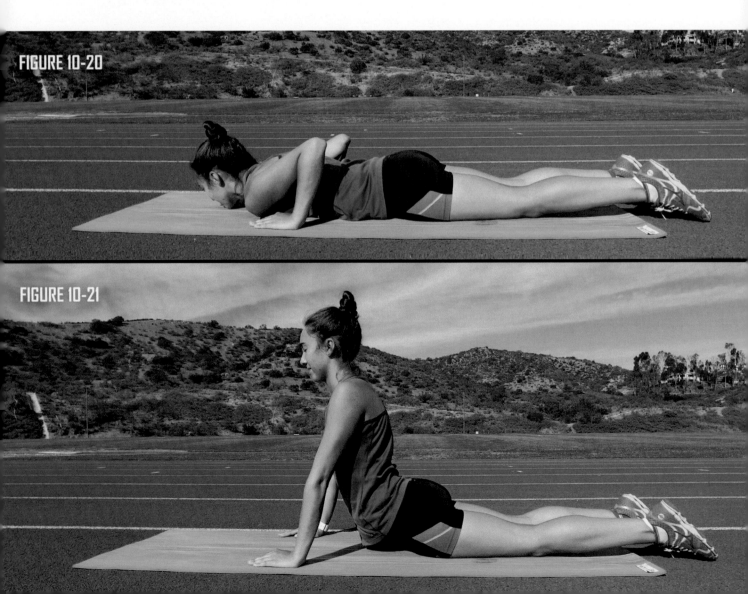

FIGURE 10-20

FIGURE 10-21

STANDING BACK
STRETCH

The **Standing Back** stretch corrects the problem of leaning forward due to tight abdominal and back muscles. It does so by stretching them into extension.

BODY POSITION

Stand with your feet shoulder width apart.

STEPS

A) Place your hands behind your back (Figure 10-22).
B) Lean backwards (Figure 10-23).
C) Hold for two seconds.
D) Return to the upright posture.
E) Repeat ten times.

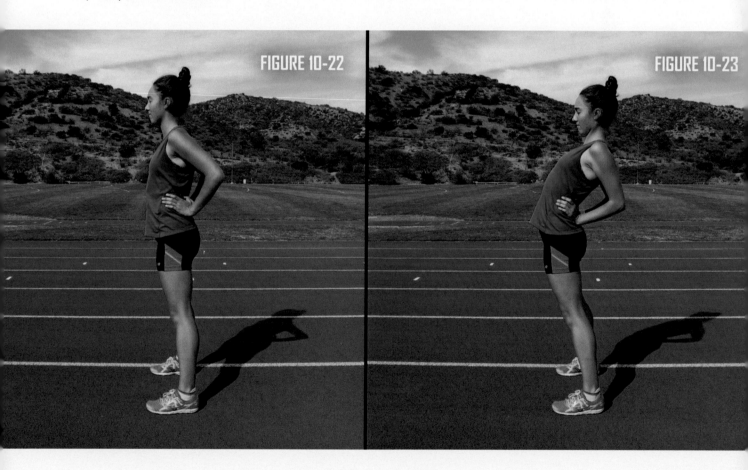

FIGURE 10-22

FIGURE 10-23

Correcting Leaning Backward

People lean backward for many reasons. The major culprits are weak abdominal muscles and a tight lower back. Both of these conditions lead to inefficient race walking style, but more importantly they can lead to injuries and lower back pain.

While it may take a while to correct this problem, it is time well spent, because the benefits from the following exercises will not only help your race walking, but also help you walk better in your daily life.

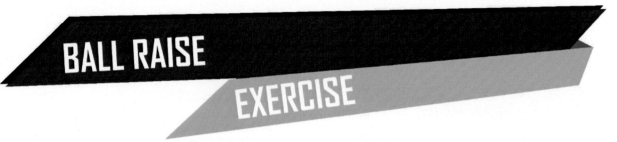

BALL RAISE EXERCISE

This exercise strengthens the abdominals and shoulders, helping to prevent leaning backwards.

BODY POSITION

Hold an exercise ball in front of your body and below your waist (Figure 10-24).

STEPS

A) Exhale while you raise the ball to the height of your forehead, making sure to keep your back straight (Figure 10-25); Tighten your abdominals as you raise the ball.
B) Continue to exhale as you hold the ball in place for 2-3 seconds.
C) Inhale while you slowly lower the ball to your waist.
D) Repeat 15 to 20 times.

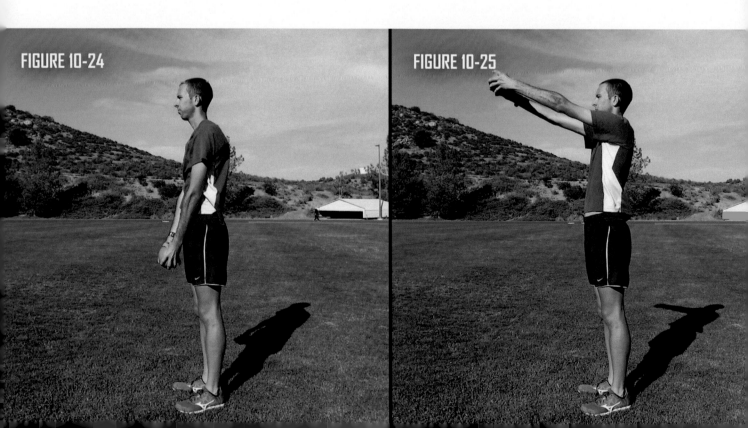

FIGURE 10-24

FIGURE 10-25

TRADITIONAL STOMACH CRUNCHES
EXERCISE

Use the **Traditional Stomach Crunches** as a very basic method of strengthening your abdominal muscles without overly stressing your back to help prevent a backward lean.

BODY POSITION

Start by lying down on a firm surface. Bend your knees and bring both feet toward your buttocks, so that your legs form a triangle with the ground (Figure 10-26).

STEPS

A) Place your hands across your chest and exhale while curling upward with your chin tucked against your chest; Roll your upper body off the ground (as much as eight inches), pressing your lower back to the ground as you curl (Figure 10-27).
B) Hold for three seconds.
C) Inhale while reversing your movements and lowering your body to its original position.
D) Repeat the exercise as many times as possible (up to a maximum of 100 crunches), but only as long as you can maintain good technique.

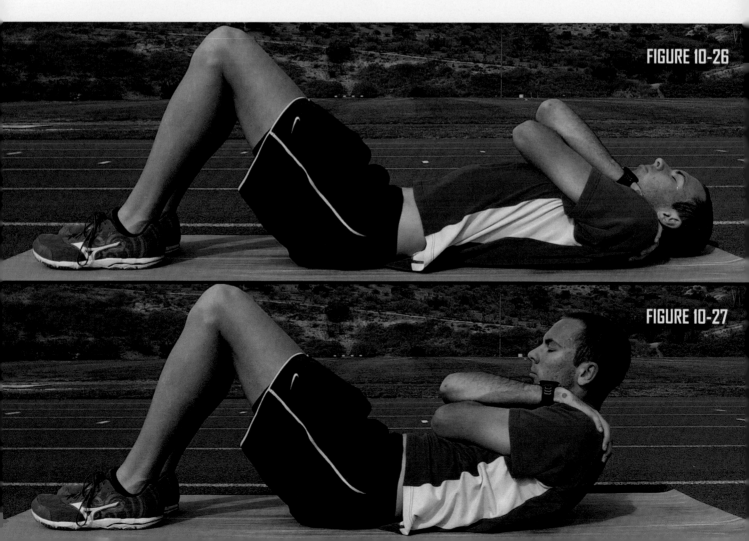

FIGURE 10-26

FIGURE 10-27

BICYCLE EXERCISE

The **Bicycle Exercise** adds a twisting motion to the **Traditional Stomach Crunch** to increase greater range of abdominal muscles.

BODY POSITION

Lay down on a firm surface.

STEPS

A) Touch your left elbow to your right knee, lifting your torso up as you do (Figure 10-28).
B) Simultaneously lower your raised elbow and knee while raising the opposite knee and elbow (Figure 10-29).
C) Repeat the exercise 25 times.

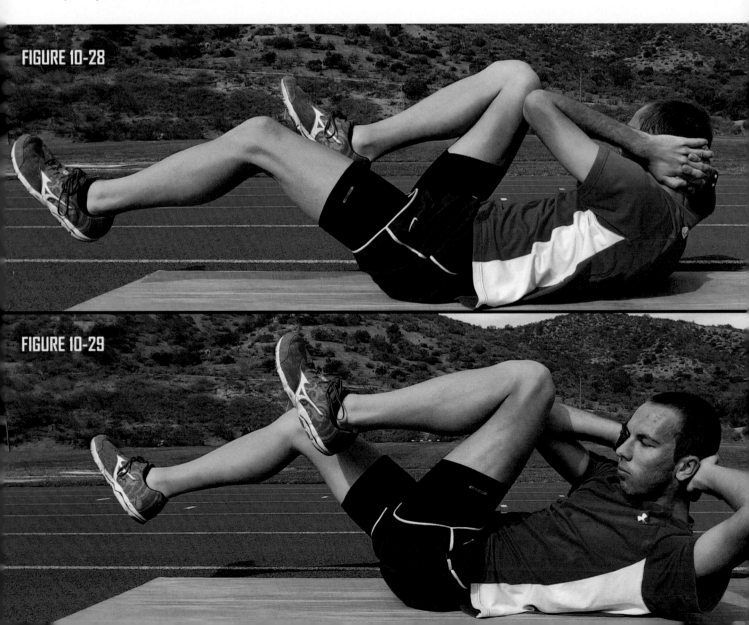

FIGURE 10-28

FIGURE 10-29

UPPER BACK
STRETCH

The **Upper Back** stretch allows you to get more comfortable posture and remove your backward lean by stretching your upper back.

BODY POSITION

Wrap your hands around a pole, standing far enough back that your arms are straight. Place your feet comfortably so you maintain balance.

STEPS

A) Lean backward, feeling the stretch through your upper back (Figure 10-30).
B) Hold for ten seconds.
C) Return to a standing position.
D) Repeat three times.

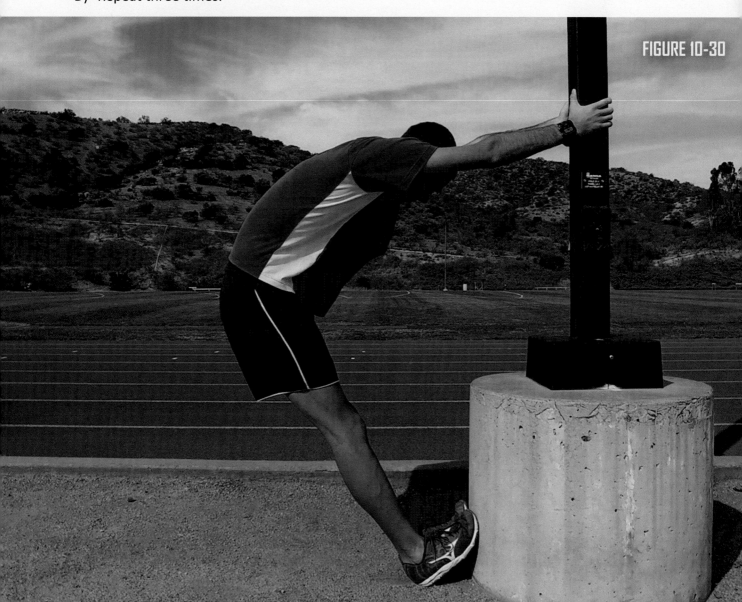

FIGURE 10-30

KNEES TO CHEST
STRETCH

This is a comfortable way to stretch the lower back and remediate a backward leaning posture.

BODY POSITION

Lie down on your back and place your hands just before the hamstring/ knee insertion point (Figure 10-31).

STEPS

Pull your knees towards your chest and hold for 30 seconds (Figure 10-32) and repeat 5 times.

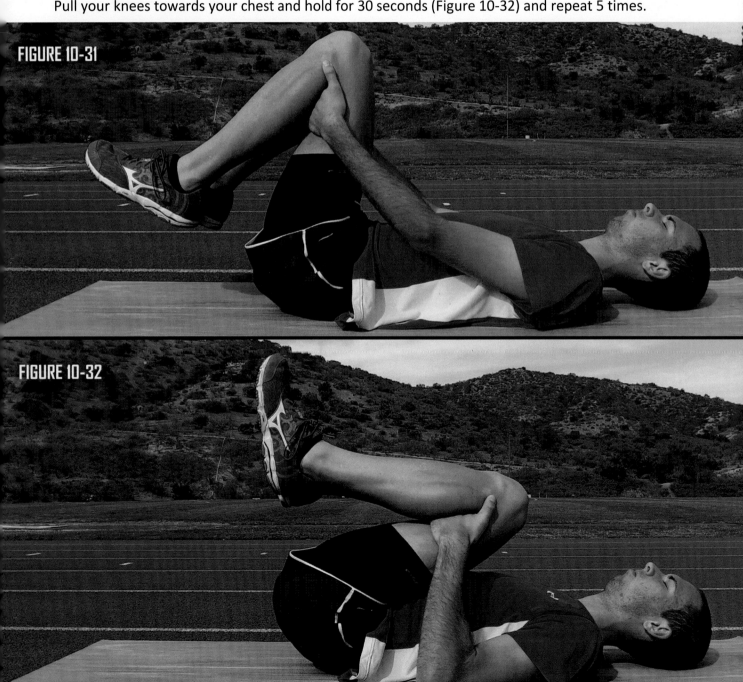

FIGURE 10-31

FIGURE 10-32

PRAYER STRETCH

A simple, comfortable way to stretch the lower back and help remediate a backward lean in your posture.

BODY POSITION

Kneel on the floor, with your knees hip width apart.

STEPS

A) Use your hands for support.
B) Lower your head.
C) Slide back to a seated position with your buttocks on your heels.
D) Stretch forward, reaching out with your hands (Figure 10-33).
E) Hold for 30 seconds.
F) You can alternate by rotating your hands to each side.
G) Repeat five times.

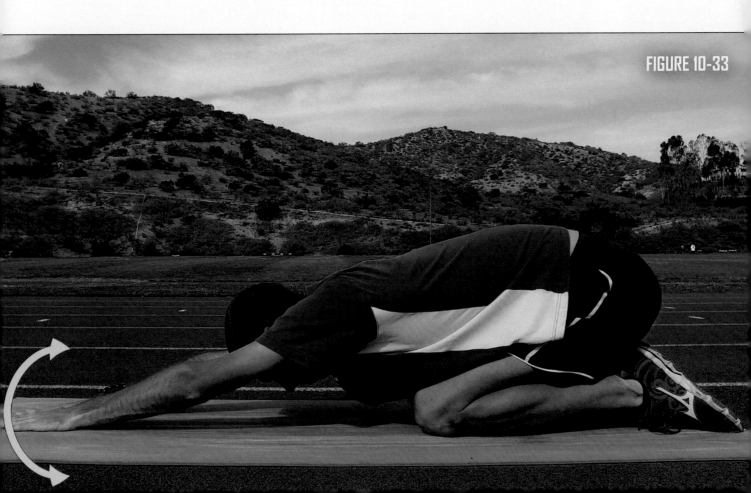

FIGURE 10-33

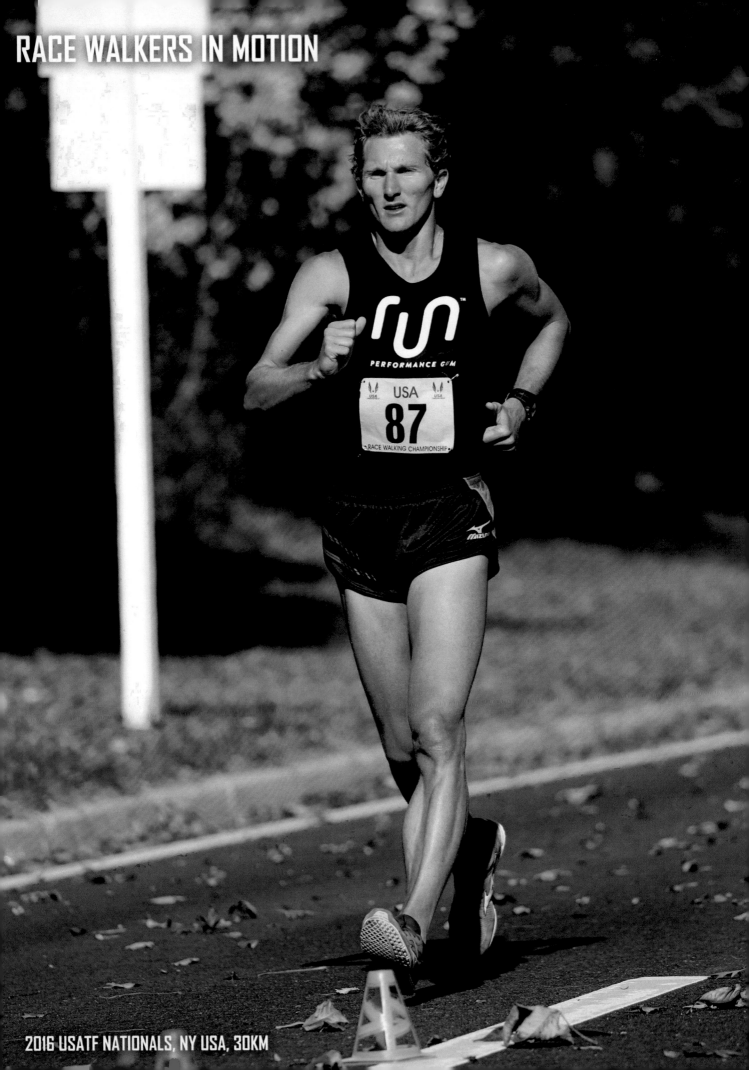

RACE WALKERS IN MOTION

2016 USATF NATIONALS, NY USA, 30KM

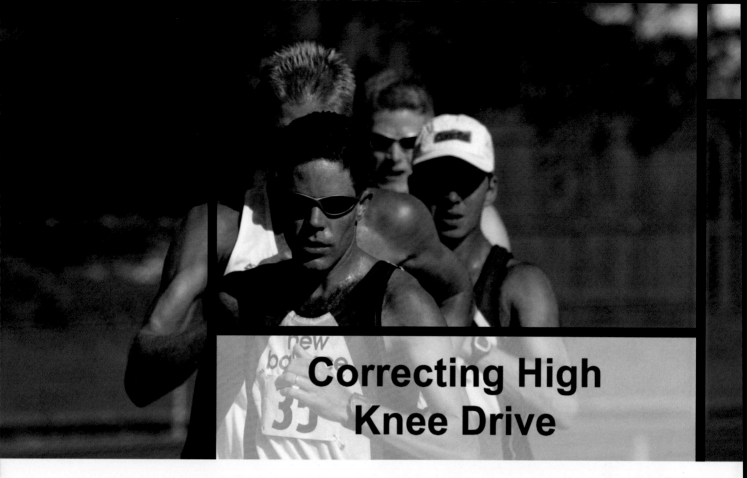

Correcting High Knee Drive

Walking with a high knee drive is fraught with problems. While you may be walking with one foot in contact with the ground at all times, a high knee drive may make you appear to lose contact. Even if you are not getting disqualified, you still need to be concerned about wasted energy by moving your leg up and down further than necessary. The leg is approximately 15 to 20 percent of the body's weight. Lifting it higher than necessary, approximately 20,000 times during a 20km race, wastes a lot of energy. Additionally, a high knee drive, gives you the appearance of running instead of having a fluid movement. Your head may also bounce up and down, creating an added jarring motion in your stride and potentially increasing your chance of injury.

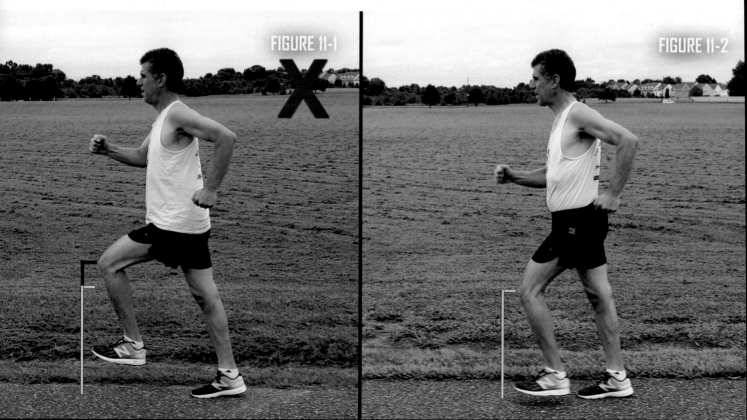

FIGURE 11-1

FIGURE 11-2

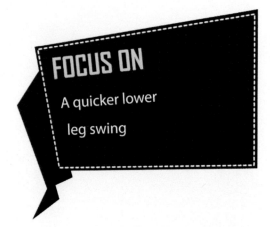

FOCUS ON

A quicker lower
leg swing

Instead of driving your leg forward with the top of your leg leading the way, once the knee passes under the torso focus on swinging the lower leg and foot as fast as possible until your heel strikes the ground.

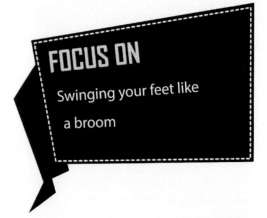

FOCUS ON

Swinging your feet like
a broom

One method to get your knees lower is to think of your swinging foot like a broom, sweeping as low to the ground as possible. Studies have shown that the higher the foot is swinging through the stride, the more likely the athlete is to get loss of contact violations.

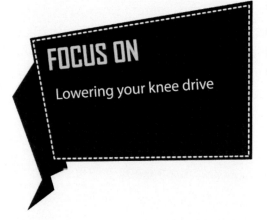

FOCUS ON

Lowering your knee drive

While it may sound obvious, to prevent a high knee drive, focus on keeping your knee low. When the leg swings forward and the knee drives upwards, it gives the appearance of loss of contact.

SCUFF WALKING DRILL

By dragging your foot along the ground, you are training your body not to drive the knee high. Once the body is accustomed to walking with low foot carriage, you can raise the foot slightly and will be race walking with improved knee drive.

BODY POSITION

Stand as you would when you are race walking.

STEPS

A) Walk slowly, swinging the foot so low that you scuff your toes on the ground as they move forward.
B) Do this for 30 to 50 meters. Do not scuff your feet for an entire lap or through a full workout.

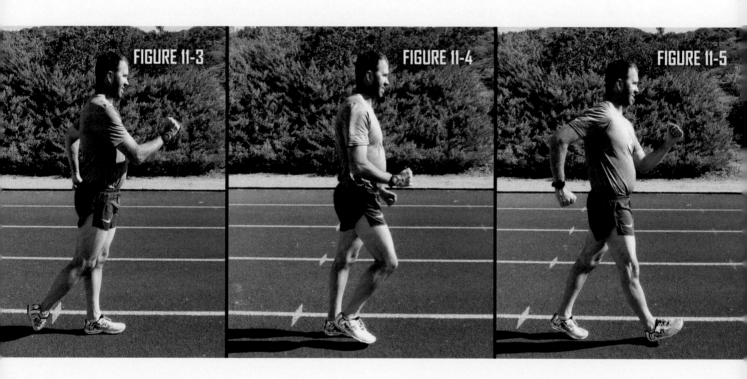

FIGURE 11-3   FIGURE 11-4   FIGURE 11-5

FOOT PLANT DRILL

One side effect of high knee drive is that you carry your foot through too high as well. By practicing the **Foot Plant** drill, you repeat the action of your foot swinging low to the ground. Really focus on foot placement when doing this drill to correct high knee drive.

See chapter 3, page 12 for steps to complete this drill.

HIP FLEXOR - LUNGE FORWARD STRETCH

Tight hip flexors make it difficult to maintain a long stride behind the torso, due to the associated lack of hip rotation. Therefore, the rear foot lifts off the ground prematurely, often causing a high knee drive. To prevent this, make sure that your hip flexors allow a greater range of motion.

See chapter 9, page 104 for steps to complete this drill.

ADVANCED HIP FLEXOR STRETCH

In addition to the **Hip Flexor** stretch, this advanced stretch may be used to further improve forward hip rotation and thus reduce high knee drive.

See chapter 9, page 106 for steps to complete this drill.

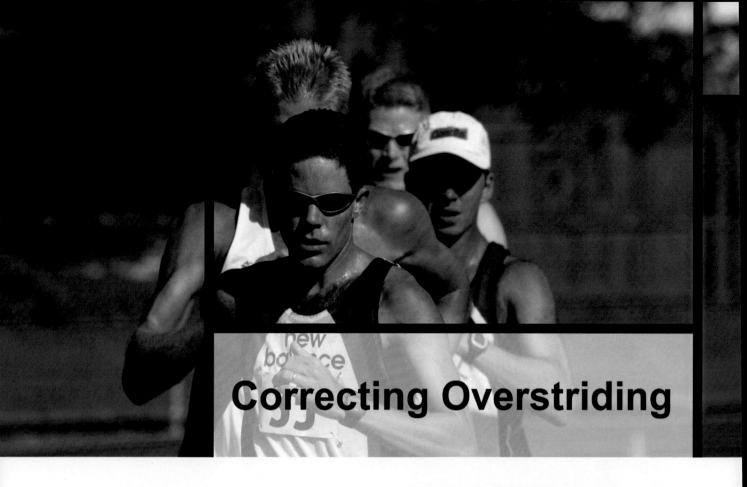

Correcting Overstriding

Overstriding in front of your body (Figure 12-1) makes it difficult to walk efficiently and can lead to the perception that you've lost contact with the ground. A tight hip flexor causes the rear foot to lift off the ground prematurely and shortens the stride where you want it the longest. In addition, overstriding may be caused due to poor arm swing or just overly zealous effort (usually when you are tired and muscling through). Observe how much better Miranda looks in Figure 12-2 where she is walking with an appropriate stride length.

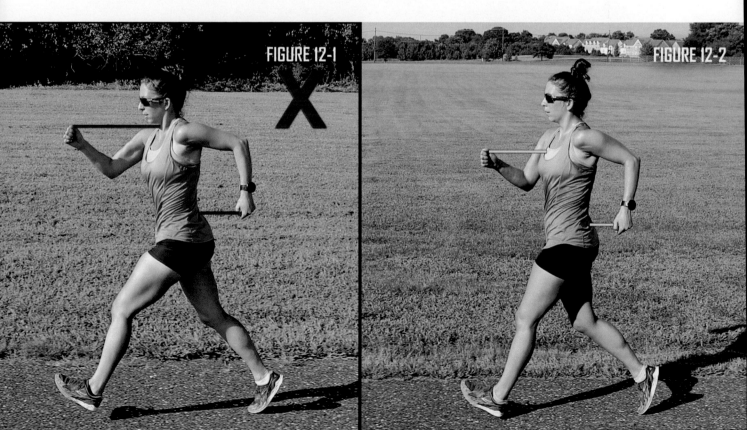

FIGURE 12-1

FIGURE 12-2

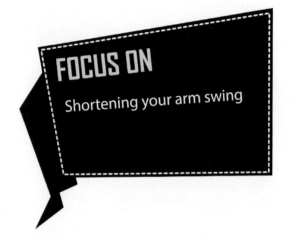

FOCUS ON

Shortening your arm swing

Work on shortening your arm swing so that the hands come back to at most 4 to 6 inches behind the hips. The arms, hips, and legs all move in rhythm and are proportional. A decrease in arm swing should reduce your stride length. Some people incorrectly profess that the peak of the upper arm's range of motion should be when the upper arm is parallel to the ground. Instead, the peak of the upper arm's range of motion should come when the upper arm swings backward coming up to an angle of 20-30 degrees (See chapter 4, page 20.)

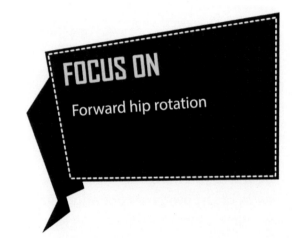

FOCUS ON

Forward hip rotation

Often overstriding in front of the body is caused by a lack of forward hip rotation. Concentrate on driving your hip forward to reduce the percentage of your stride that is in front of your torso.

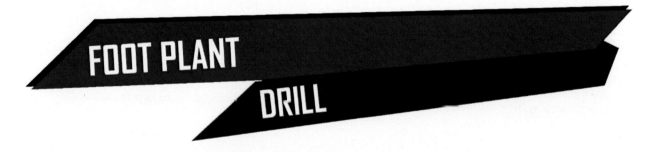

FOOT PLANT DRILL

Part of the problem with overstriding is that your foot dangles out in front of the body, neither pushing nor pulling your body forward. If you place your foot just in front of your body, your stride becomes more efficient.

See chapter 3, page 12 for steps to complete this drill.

HIP FLEXOR - LUNGE FORWARD
STRETCH

Any stretch or drill that improves the range of motion of the hip flexors will reduce overstriding.

See chapter 9, page 104 for steps to complete this drill.

ADVANCED HIP FLEXOR
STRETCH

Any stretch or drill that improves the range of motion of the hip flexors will reduce overstriding.

See chapter 9, page 106 for steps to complete this drill.

LONG STRIDES - LONG ARMS
DRILL

Any stretch or drill that improves the range of motion of the hip flexors will reduce overstriding.

See chapter 5, page 47 for steps to complete this drill.

QUICK STEPS
DRILL

Any of the **Quick Steps** drills can be added to your routine to correct overstriding. If you choose one, the **Quick Steps – Hands Behind Back** drill is best. If you have time, do the other varieties as well as they will also improve your turnover rate.

See chapter 7, page 86 for steps to complete this drill.

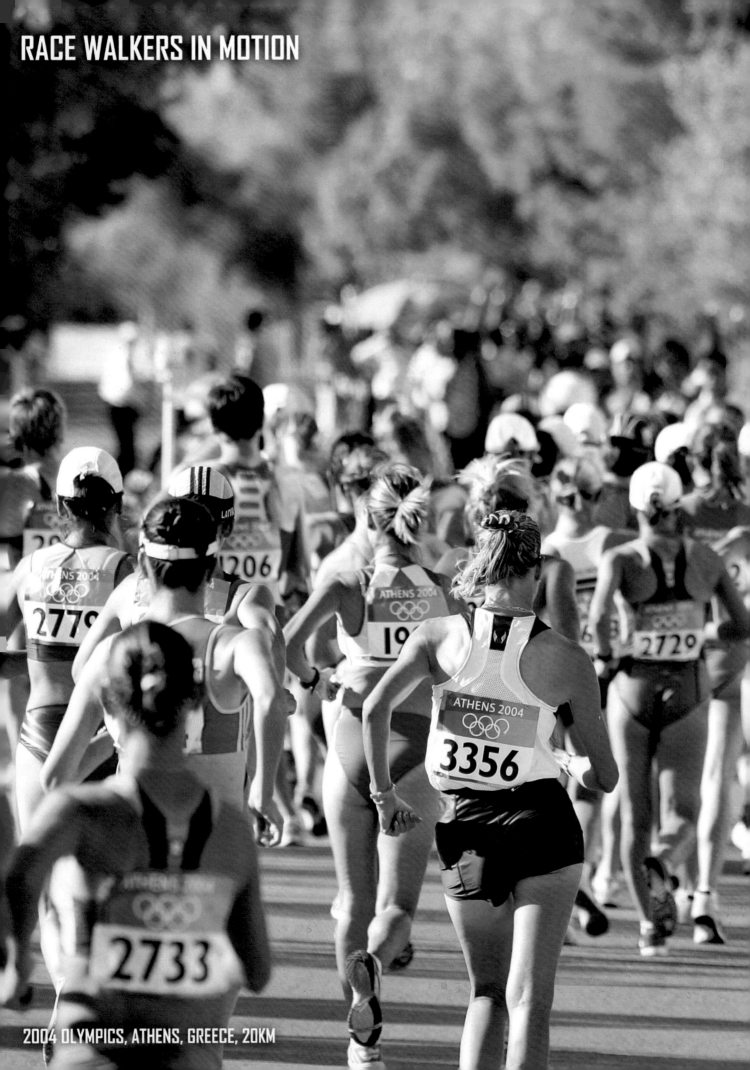

2004 OLYMPICS, ATHENS, GREECE, 20KM

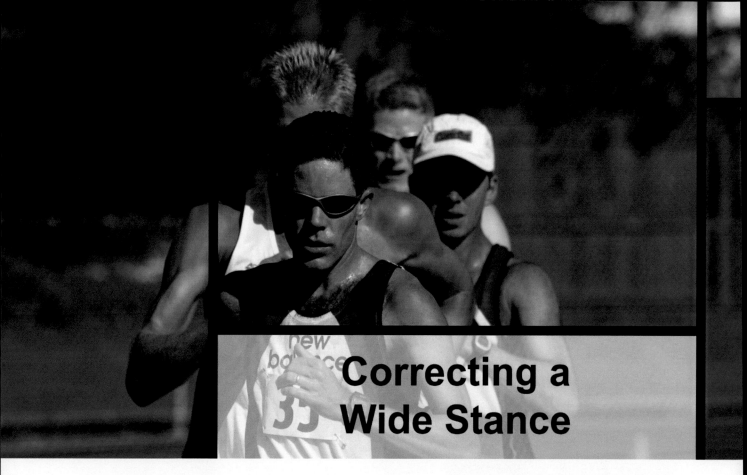

Correcting a
Wide Stance

When pedestrians walk quickly, they rarely change their technique; they merely walk with a more exaggerated stride at a faster cadence (Figure 13-1). This gets them only so far or fast. Race walkers (Figure 13-2), in contrast, change many aspects of their stride, most notably adding a forward drive of the hip as the leg swings forward. Most race walkers who walk with a wide stance do so because they do not rotate their hips forward and therefore inward. Since the hip cannot move forward in a straight line, it must rotate inward as it rotates forward. As it does, it causes the foot to land along a straight line.

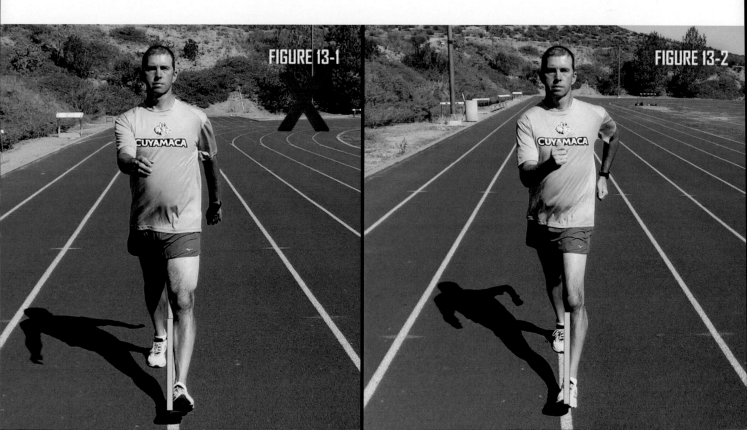

FIGURE 13-1   FIGURE 13-2

To correct a wide stance, you can perform any of the corrections for incorrect hip rotation as taught in chapter 8.

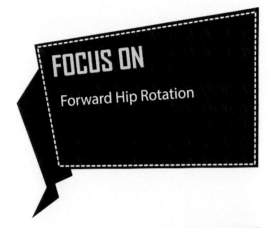

FOCUS ON

Forward Hip Rotation

It may seem that we keep repeating hips, hips, and more hips, but they are key to many problems with race walking technique. If your feet are not landing in a straight line, it is probably due to a lack of forward hip rotation. When the hip rotates forward, it also rotates inward, causing the feet to land in a straight line. Concentrate on driving your hip forward and your foot placement naturally straightens out.

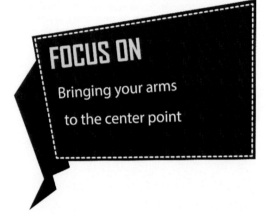

FOCUS ON

Bringing your arms
to the center point

Focus on bringing your arms to the center point in front of your body in line with your sternum as shown in Figures 13-3 & 13-4. Synchronize the placement of your feet, so that they land "underneath" your hands.

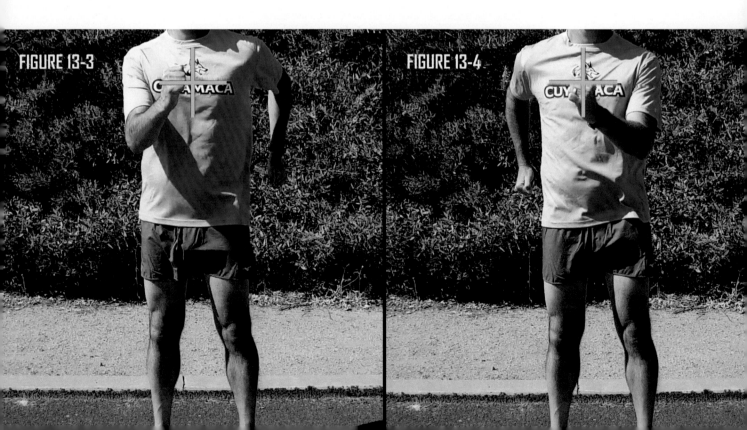

FIGURE 13-3

FIGURE 13-4

STRAIGHT LINE WALKING
DRILL

When trying to correct a wide stance, one can encourage the hips to rotate forward by walking along a straight line. It is important to note that your footfalls land in a straight line as a result of proper hip rotation and not just forcing your feet to land along a straight line without any rotation of the hips.

See chapter 9, page 98 for steps to complete this drill.

FOOT PLANT
DRILL

The **Foot Plant** drill focuses your attention on the proper way to place your foot down.

See chapter 3, page 12 for steps to complete this drill.

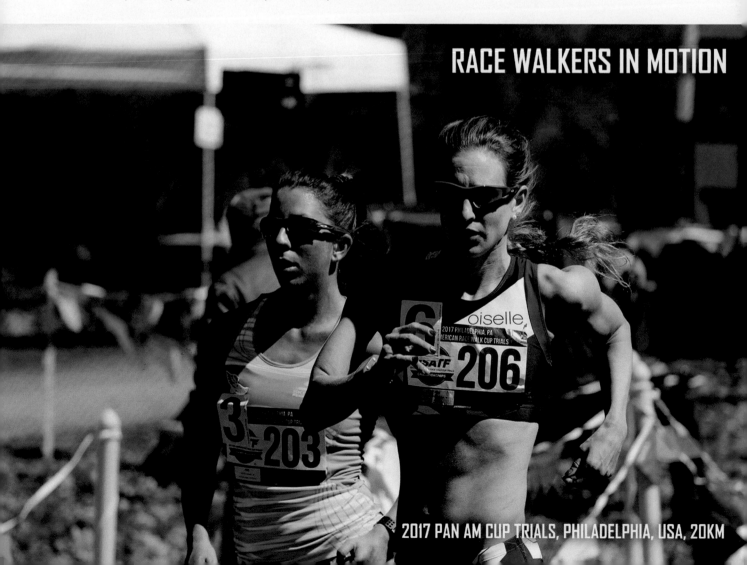

RACE WALKERS IN MOTION

2017 PAN AM CUP TRIALS, PHILADELPHIA, USA, 20KM

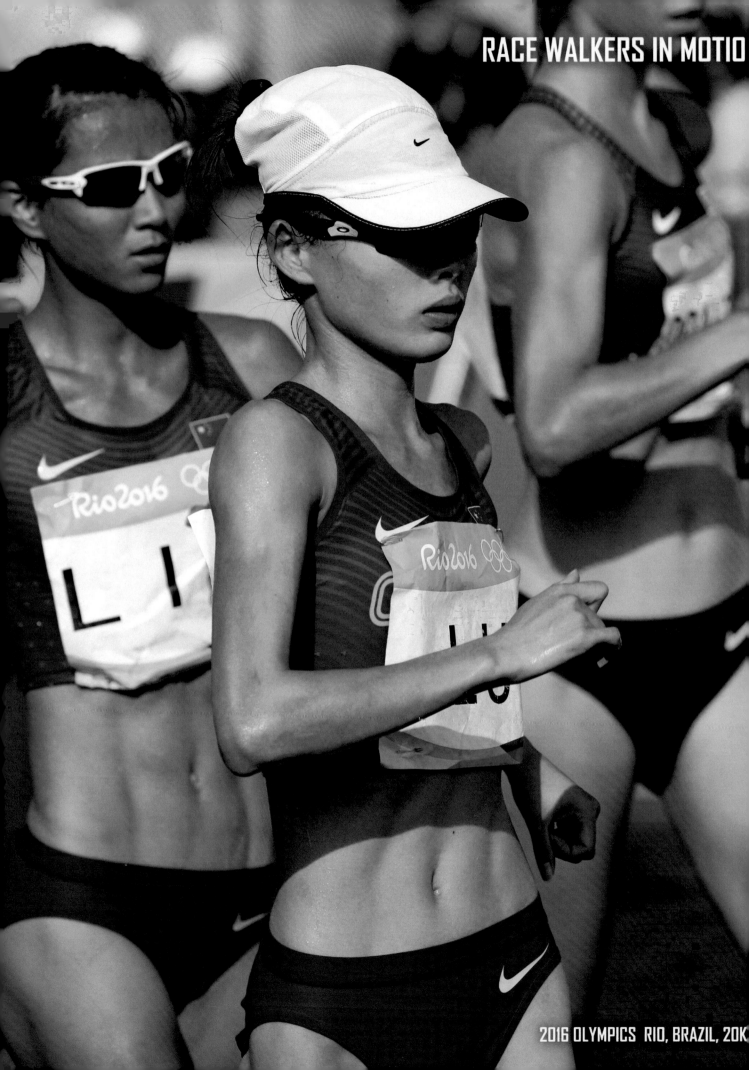

2016 OLYMPICS RIO, BRAZIL, 20K

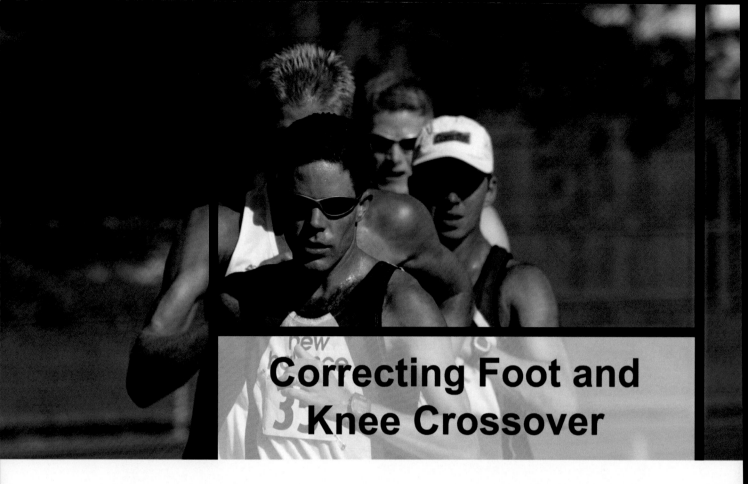

Correcting Foot and Knee Crossover

While it's fairly rare to see a race walker cross one foot over the other (Figures 14-1 & 14-2), it does happen. In fact, we used to speak of it hypothetically until at a recent clinic, a young beginning race walker who lacked the muscle control to keep his legs and feet in line demonstrated this problem as part of his stride. While there are no specific exercises to correct this, use the following two visualizations to correct crossover problems.

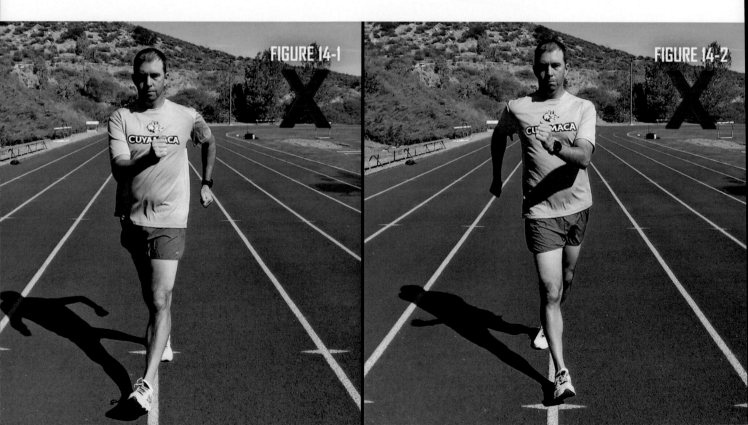

FIGURE 14-1

FIGURE 14-2

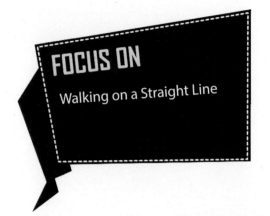

FOCUS ON
Walking on a Straight Line

Focus on walking on a straight line. If you are crossing over the line, then you are wasting effort to the side instead of driving yourself forward.

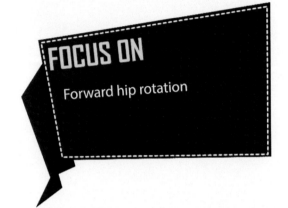

FOCUS ON
Forward hip rotation

Swiveling your hips around the axis that runs through the middle of your body is **NOT** desirable. Hip motion must be primarily forward. So consciously extend your hip forward as the leg swings forward. Minimize the inward rotation.

STRAIGHT LINE WALKING DRILL

Since foot and knee crossover is largely due to lack of muscle control, walking along a straight line refocuses your technique.

See chapter 9, page 98 for steps to complete this drill.

SIDE STRAIGHT LEG RAISE EXERCISE

Strengthening the abductors in conjunction with the *Lower Side Straight Leg Raise* exercise increases your control as you place your foot on the ground.

See chapter 9, page 102 for steps to complete this drill.

LOWER SIDE STRAIGHT LEG RAISE
EXERCISE

Strengthening the adductors, which in conjunction with the **Side Straight Leg Raise** exercise, increases your control as you place your foot on the ground.

See chapter 9, page 103 for steps to complete this drill.

FOOT PLANT
DRILL

The **Foot Plant** drill focuses your attention on the proper way to place your foot down.

See chapter 3, page 12 for steps to complete this drill.

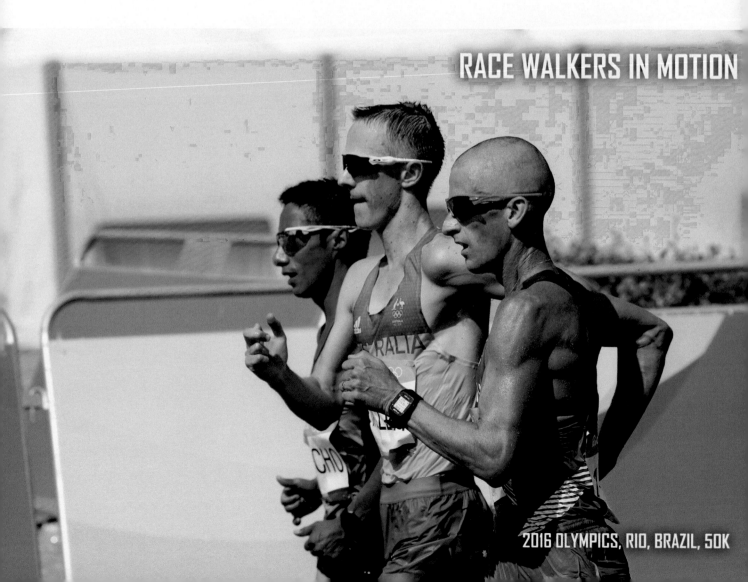

RACE WALKERS IN MOTION

2016 OLYMPICS, RIO, BRAZIL, 50K

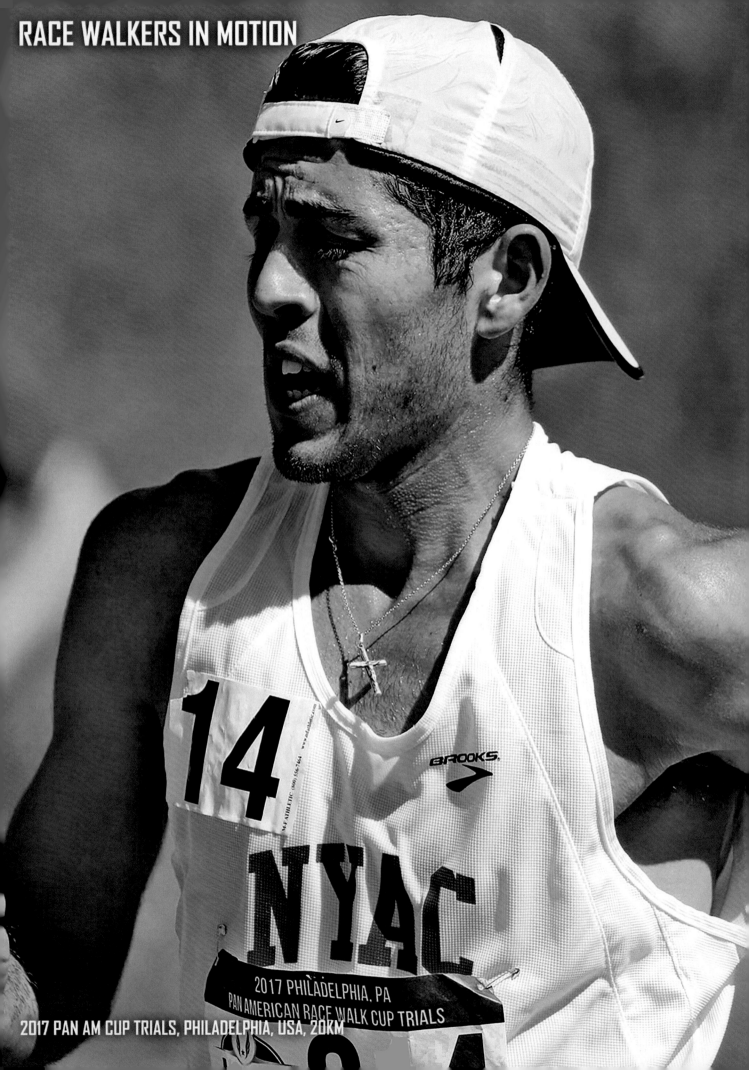

2017 PAN AM CUP TRIALS, PHILADELPHIA, USA, 20KM

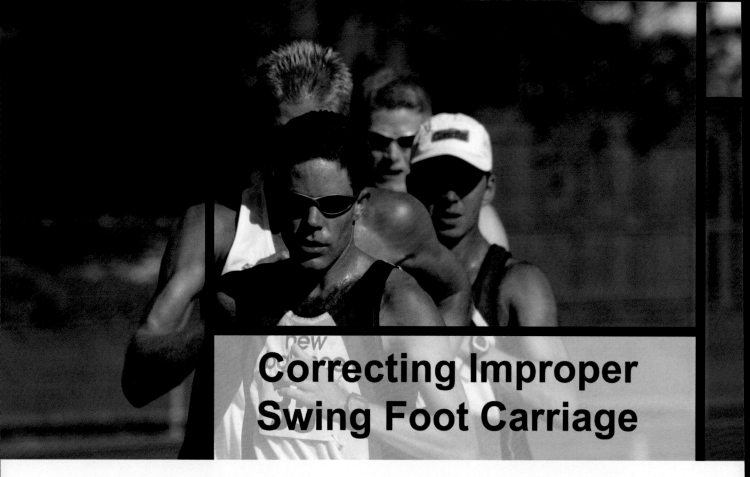

Correcting Improper Swing Foot Carriage

A very common problem for race walkers is excessive rotation of the swing foot as it travels forward after push off. It can be caused by a wide variety of muscle imbalances, tightness in many areas, or both. It is most likely to be a weakness or tightness in the hip abductor, hip flexor, quadriceps, hamstrings, or anterior of your shins. A coach can best assess the exact cause and can recommend the specific exercise to correct it.

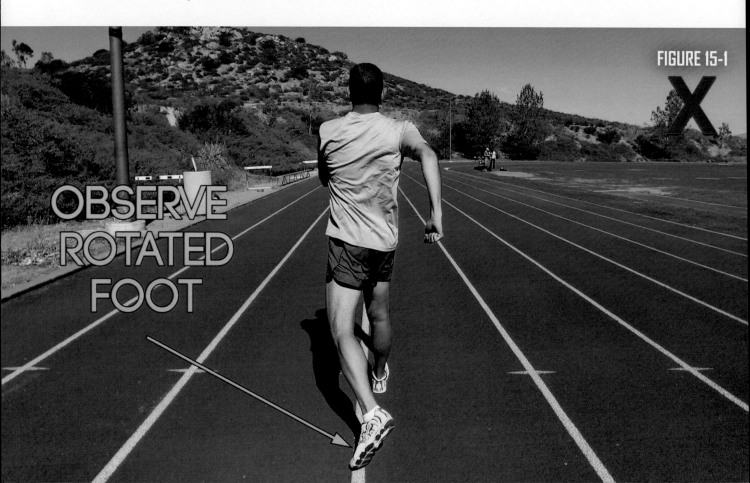

FIGURE 15-1

OBSERVE ROTATED FOOT

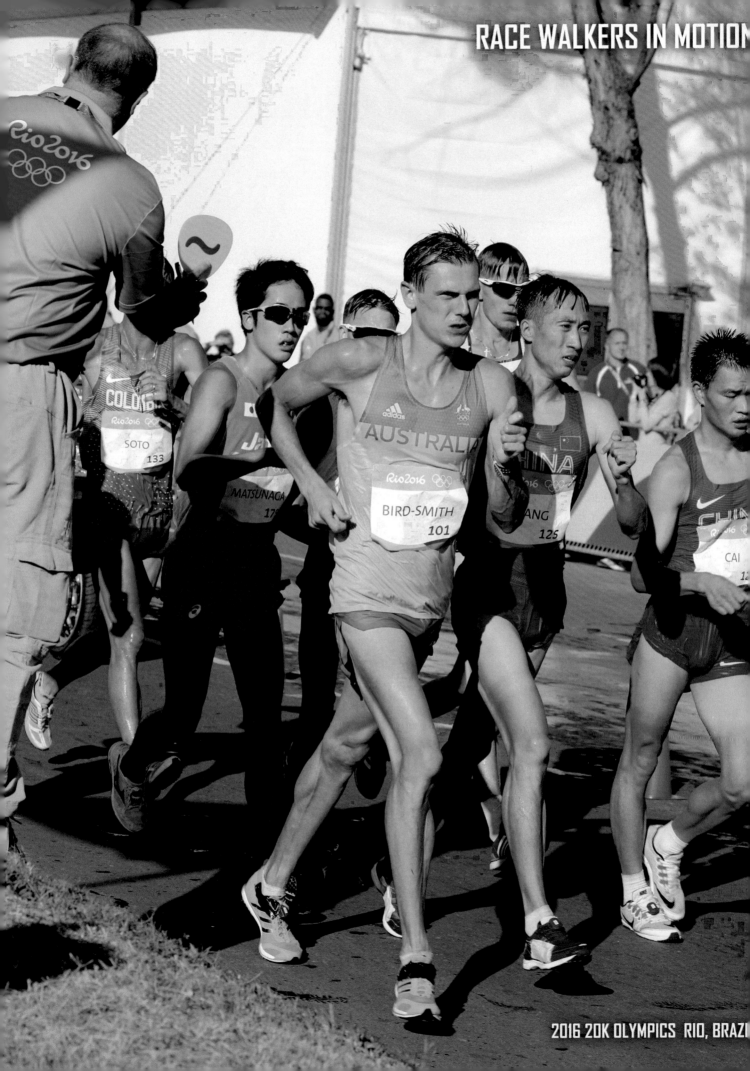

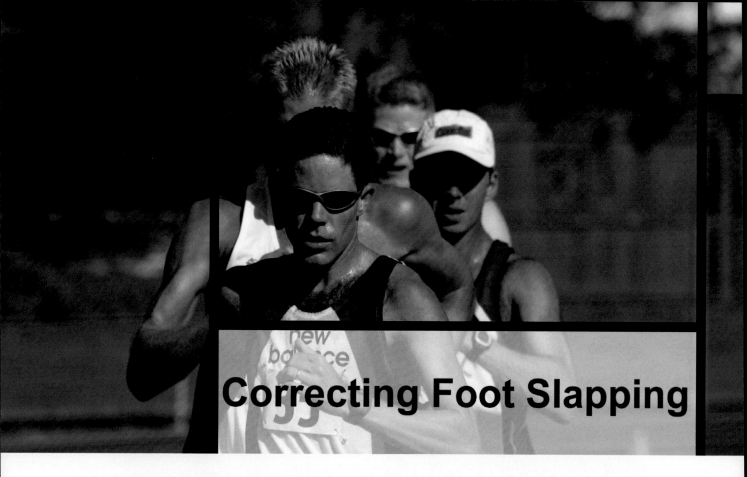

Correcting Foot Slapping

Some walkers can glide by you without your hearing a single footstep. They do this by rolling through the stride, first landing with the toe pointed as the heel makes contact with the ground and then gradually progressing forward as the toe lowers. In contrast, some walkers land flatfooted. This makes it almost impossible to land with a straightened leg. Other walkers land with a toe pointed, but flatten too quickly. This can make a you walk as if you have square tires.

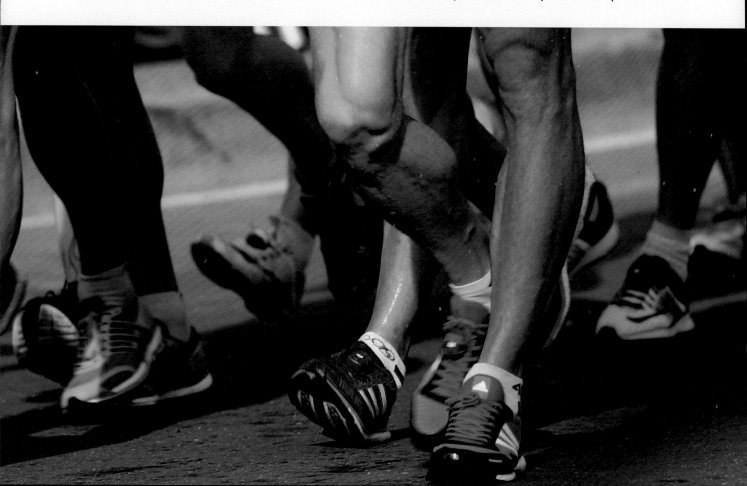

To fix either of these problems you should practice a subset of the drills, stretches and exercises we've already introduced for fixing a bent knee. They are:

FOOT PLANT DRILL

Details can be found in chapter 3, page 12.

WALK ON HEELS DRILL

Details can be found in chapter 5, page 49.

WALKING ON YOUR TOES DRILL

Details can be found in chapter 5, page 51.

CALF RAISE EXERCISE

Details can be found in chapter 5, page 52.

TOE RAISE EXERCISE

Details can be found in chapter 5, page 50.

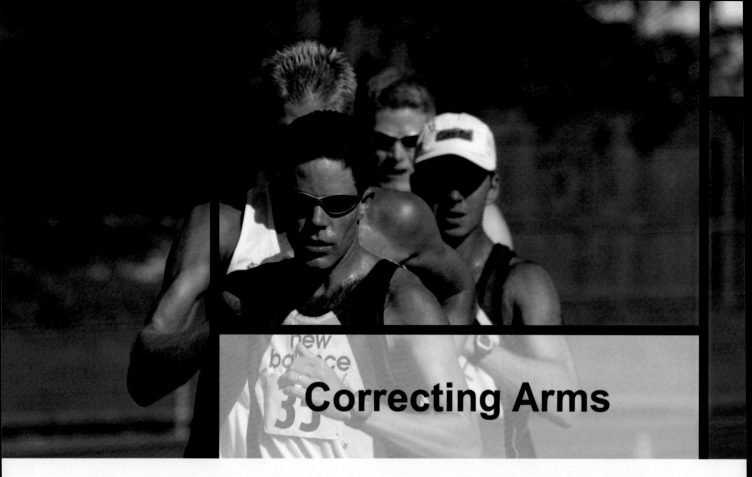

Correcting Arms

There are many ways to vary from the ideal arm carriage. Fortunately, by focusing on the correct technique we can fix many of the errors. Let's start by looking at good and bad arm carriage. Observe the walker in the middle. Her arm swing maintains a constant angle between the upper arm and lower arm as the hand traces from the middle of her chest to just behind the hip (Figure 17-2). In contrast, the walker in Figure 17-1 is swinging their arms too far in front and behind. We know it's too far because their wrist is in front of their ankle. Likewise, the walker to in Figure 17-3 also isn't swinging her arms through a far enough range of motion and thus limits their hip rotation and stride length.

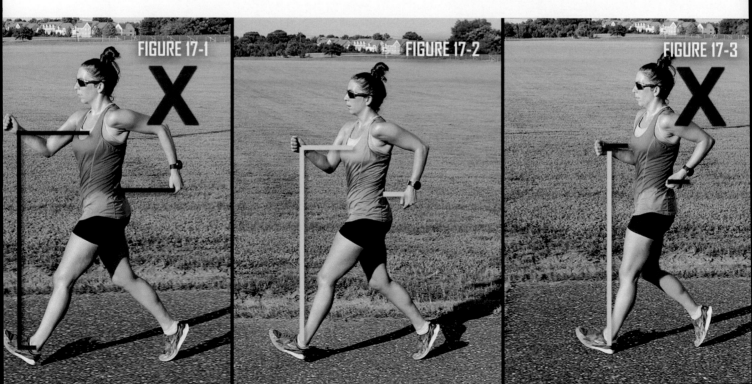

FIGURE 17-1

FIGURE 17-2

FIGURE 17-3

Walkers also have issues maintaining a constant angle between their upper and lower arm. Observe how the left arm angle of the walker in Figure 17-5 & 17-7 increases as she swings backward and decreases as she swings forward. This is a waste of energy and the excessive motion could attract the unwanted eye of a judge. Observe the proper constant arm angle in Figures 17-4 and 17-6.

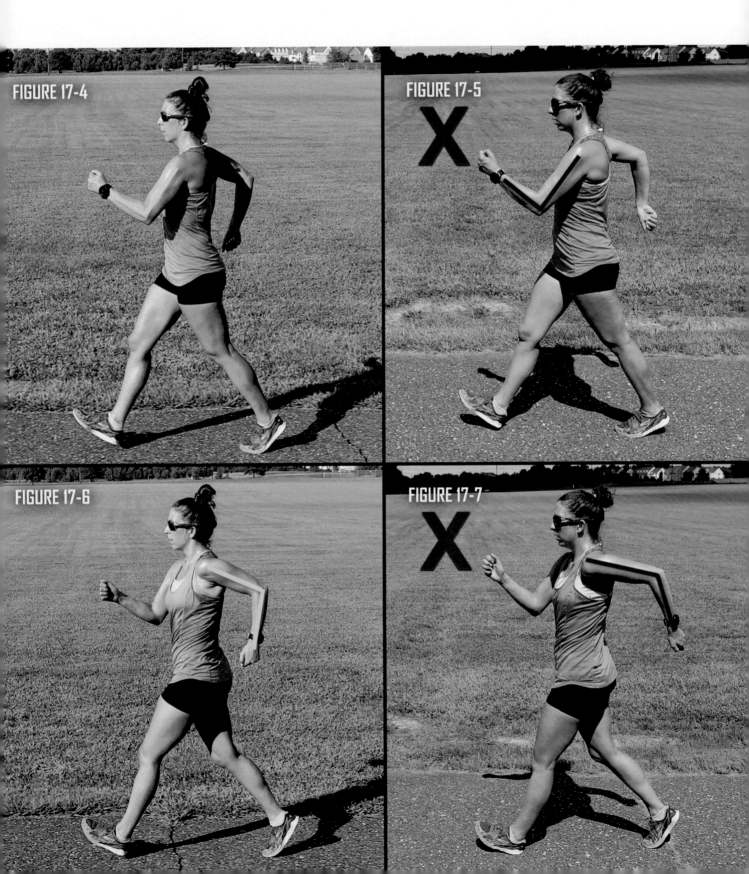

FIGURE 17-4

FIGURE 17-5

FIGURE 17-6

FIGURE 17-7

Observing walker's from the side gives a very two dimensional representation. Observe walkers from the front. It's important to make sure the arms are not robotic as shown in the walker in Figure 17-8 or crossing over too much as with the walker in Figure 17-10. Moving directly across the body or bringing the arm forward too straight inhibits forward hip rotation. Observe the proper arm swing in Figure 17-9.

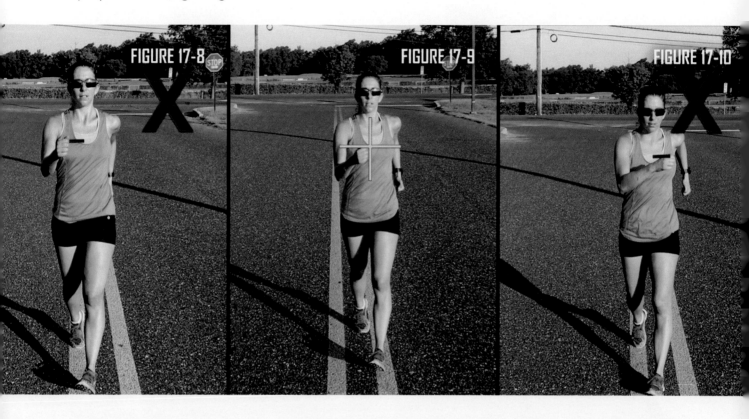

We can also fine tune the arm carriage in other ways. Look how the walker in Figure 17-12 has his arms at an angle away from the torso. This is a waste of energy. Instead, you should look more like the walker in Figure 17-11.

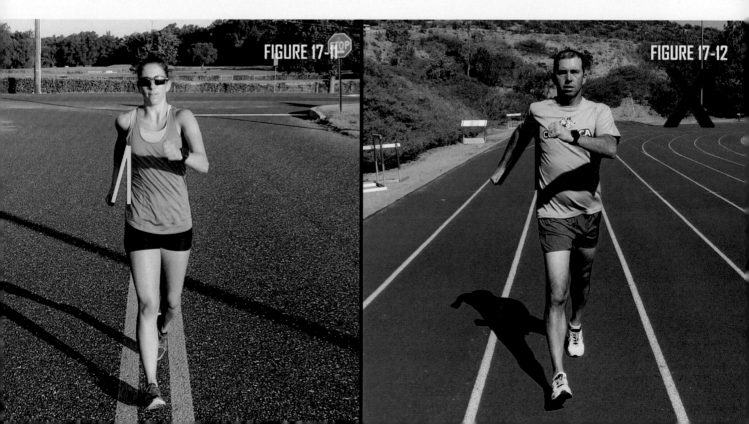

Fortunately, the cures are basically the same for all these ailments. The following focus tips can be practiced while walking or in front of a mirror.

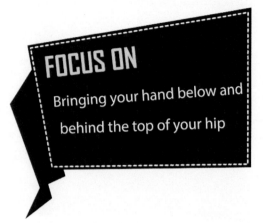

Bringing your hand back below and behind the hip is essential to achieve proper arm motion, as well as to make it easier to reach forward with your hips. If your hands do not reach back far enough, your hands will not come forward to the proper position. In addition, your hip drive is diminished. To increase the range of motion through which your arms and hands travel, increase the angle between your upper and lower arm. To decrease the range of motion through which your arms and hands travel, decrease the angle between your upper and lower arm.

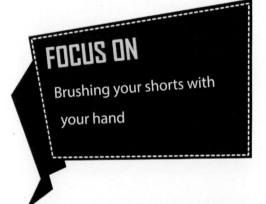

When swinging your arms forward and back, you should not swing them far from the side of your torso. If you hold your arms too far out, you waste energy supporting the weight of your arm. To get your hands and arms closer to the proper position, brush your shorts lightly with your hand.

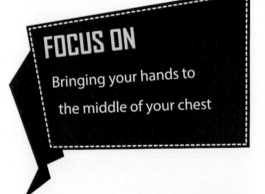

Many walkers violate this concept on both sides of the imaginary line across your chest. While there is some variation in the ending height of the forward arm swing, a good goal for the point of the arc is your chest line. If your hands are swinging above the line, then increase the angle that your forearm makes with your upper arm. In contrast, if your hands aren't swinging high enough, then decrease the angle your forearm makes with your upper arm.

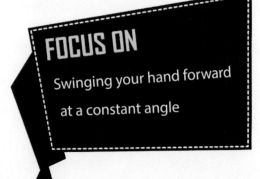

The arm swing should maintain a constant angle between the forearm and upper arm. Do not pump your arm as it swings forward and back. Resist the temptation to close the angle on the upswing and open the angle on the downswing. If you are lucky enough to attend one of our clinics, you can try out our custom arm braces to help you get the proper feel for arm swing.

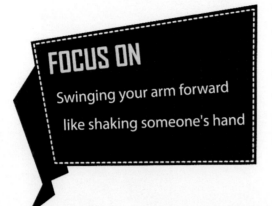
When you reach forward to shake someone's hand, your hand moves forward on an arc from the side of your hip to cross the front of your body. It should do the same in race walking. The only difference is that when you shake someone's hand, your arm angle changes, whereas in race walking the arm angle remains constant.

BICEPS STRETCH

The *Biceps* stretch is useful because, while race walkers do not pump their biceps muscles during race walking, they do use them to hold the arm at approximately a 90-degree angle while they walk. Go for a long enough walk and your biceps will get tight.

BODY POSITION

Stand up with your feet shoulder width apart.

STEPS

A) Place your hands together, behind your back, with your palms together.
B) Exhale while raising your arms until you feel the stretch.
C) Hold for 15 seconds.
D) Lower your hands.
E) Repeat three times.

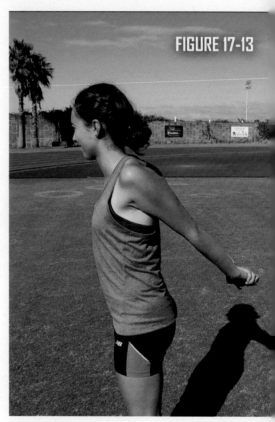

FIGURE 17-13

TRICEPS
STRETCH

Inflexible triceps muscles cause a reduction of arm angle, leading in turn to a reduction in hip rotation.

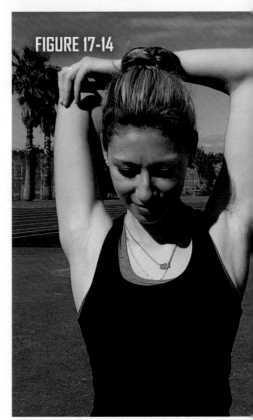

FIGURE 17-14

BODY POSITION

Stand up straight with your feet shoulder width apart.

STEPS

A) Bend your right arm back so that you touch your hand to your shoulder.
B) Grab your right elbow with your left hand.
C) Gently pull your right arm backwards.
D) Hold for 15 seconds.
E) Repeat with your other arm.

ARM SWINGS WITH ELASTIC BANDS
DRILL

Performing the **Arm Swings with Elastic Band** exercise strengthens the arms in a manner specific to race walking. While you can use weights to strengthen your biceps, triceps, etc., this drill is far more effective due to its functional nature.

See chapter 8, page 92 for steps to complete this drill.

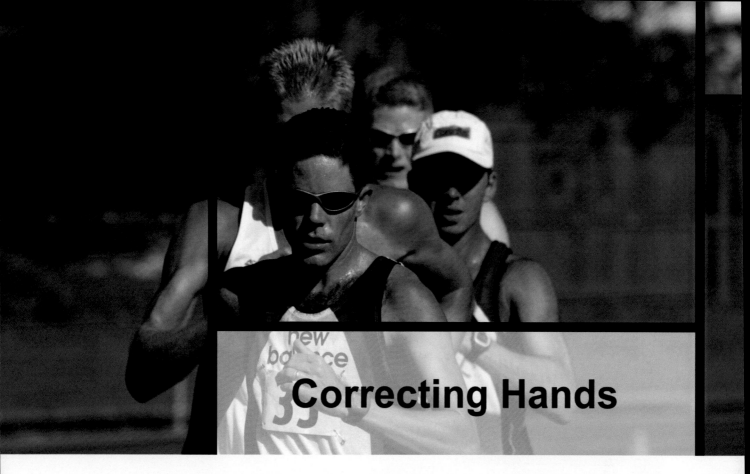

Correcting Hands

Hand carriage during race walking is quite simple. Simply keep a straight wrist with the hand in a loose fist. As your hands pass by your hips, the fingertips face the hips. However, many race walkers' hands flop all over the place (Figures 18-1 & 18-2), drawing a judge's watchful eye as well as wasting energy. There are really no exercises to help; it's primarily an issue of focus.

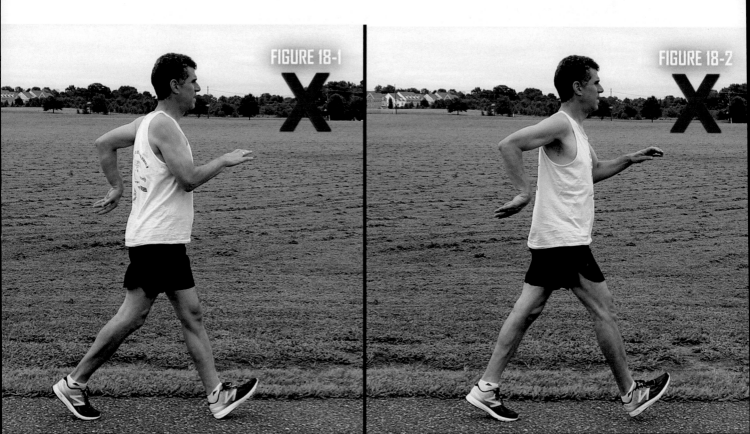

FIGURE 18-1
X

FIGURE 18-2
X

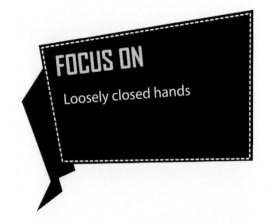

FOCUS ON

Loosely closed hands

Think about closing your hands, but do not make a fist, while you are walking.

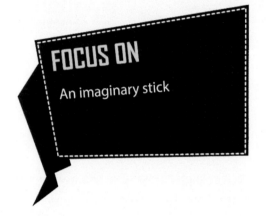

FOCUS ON

An imaginary stick

Either imagine or actually place a small stick inside your fist. Focus on keeping your hand and fingers from swaying up, down, or side to side. Coach Peña used this little trick on Andrew Hermann and it helped him walk his way onto the 2000 Sydney Olympic team.

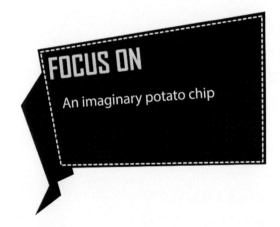

FOCUS ON

An imaginary potato chip

Too tight a fist wastes energy and leads to a tense body. Imagine that you are carrying a potato chip between your thumb and your index finger. By imagining the chip there and that you must not break it, you'll relax your hand position without letting the hand flop about.

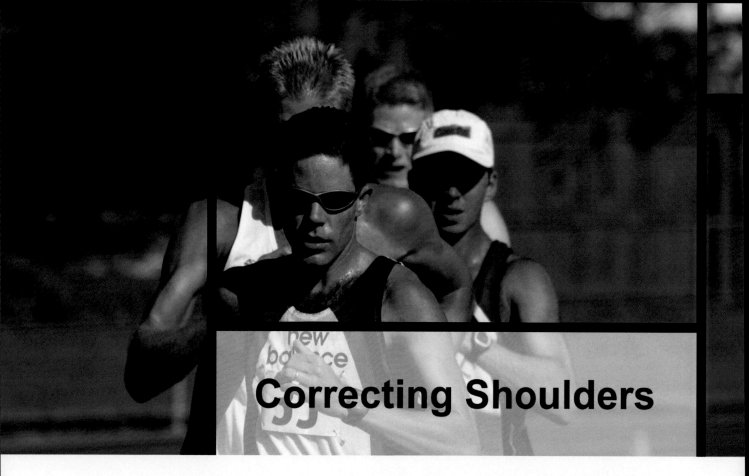

Correcting Shoulders

The most common problem with race walkers' shoulders is tightness resulting in high shoulder carriage. This also leads to a high arm carriage and due to your higher center of gravity could lead to a lifting call. In addition, tight shoulders could lead to cramps, making it difficult for you to maintain proper arm swing. Once your arms stop swinging, your hips are sure to follow. Once you lose your hips, you will be pedestrian walking the rest of the way.

Curt Clausen credits finally learning to relax his shoulders as the key to improving his arm swing and thus freeing up his hips. This technique improvement was a key factor in Clausen's bronze medal at the 1999 World Championships in Seville, Spain.

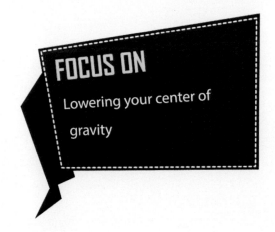

FOCUS ON

Lowering your center of gravity

Focus on a low center of gravity. When your arm swings forward and back, focus on your elbows. Keeping your elbows down lowers your center of gravity and improves your arm swing.

BACKWARD WINDMILL - STANDING DRILL

The **Reverse Windmill** Stretch is a great way to warm up the shoulders and increase your range of motion at the same time.

BODY POSITION

Slowly perform this exercise while standing with your feet approximately a shoulder width apart. Your right hand is on your right shoulder, arm relaxed, elbow toward the ground. Your left hand is on your left shoulder, but your left elbow is behind your body.

STEPS

A) Slowly raise the right elbow forward so that the arm becomes perpendicular to your body. Simultaneously, rotate the left arm backwards. Throughout the exercise as one arm rotates the other rotates similarly, but offset by 180-degrees. (Figure 19-1).

B) Continue bringing the right arm straight up, keeping your right biceps as near to your face as possible. Likewise, continue to rotate the left arm downward (Figure 19-2).

C) Slowly rotate the right arm back; It must travel outward at some point. The left arm rotates forward and starts rising (Figure 19-3).

D) Gradually rotate the left arm through a complete circle (Figure 19-4) and return to the original position while the right arm rises.

E) Repeat the rotation ten times with each arm.

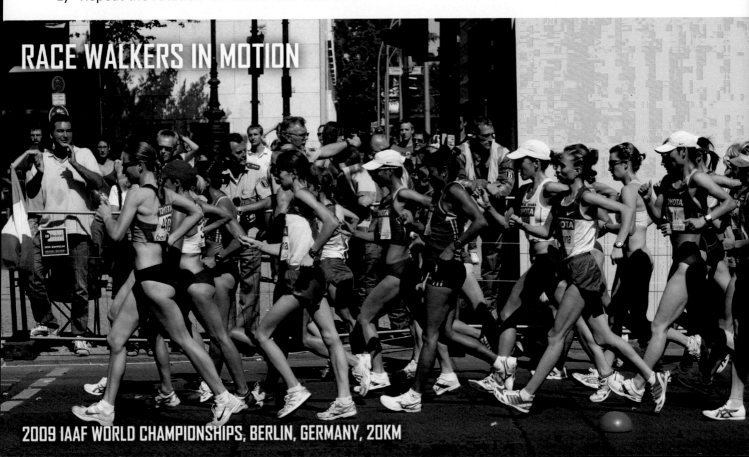

RACE WALKERS IN MOTION

2009 IAAF WORLD CHAMPIONSHIPS, BERLIN, GERMANY, 20KM

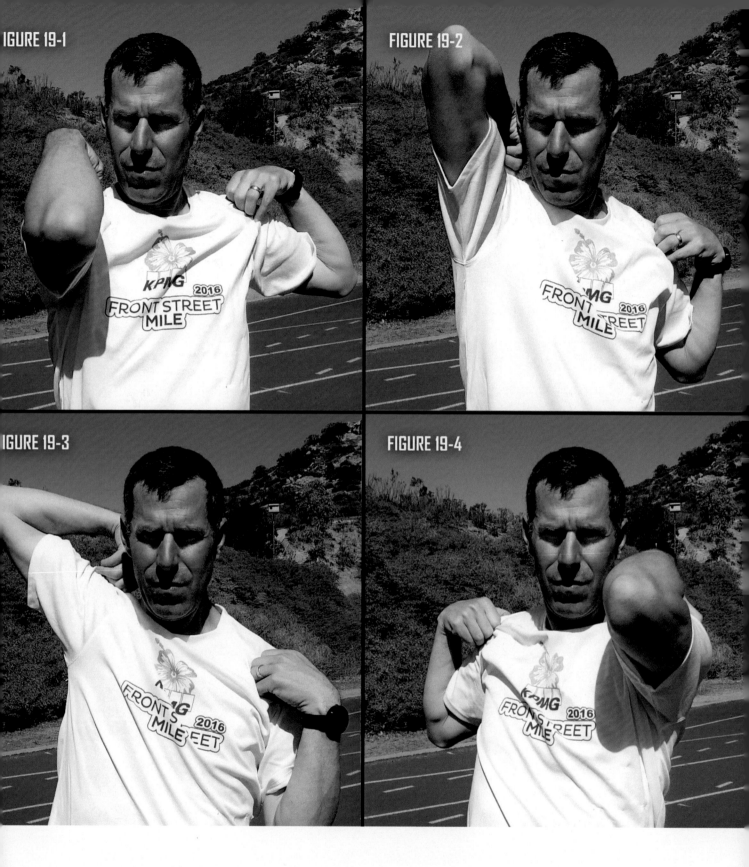

FIGURE 19-1

FIGURE 19-2

FIGURE 19-3

FIGURE 19-4

BACKWARD WINDMILL - WALKING DRILL

When the body is cold, the **Backward Windmill** drill is a great way to get blood pumping to all extremities quickly. In addition, it helps to relax and stretch the upper body (specifically targeting the shoulders), leading to a more fluid arm motion.

BODY POSITION

Stand straight up with one arm at your side and the other pointed straight up to the sky.

STEPS

A) Swing the arm at your side up and forward at the same time as you swing the pointed arm back and down allowing both arms to make circles, keeping your arm close to the side of your head as you swing it back.

B) Walk with the proper lower leg motion of race walking for 30 meters.

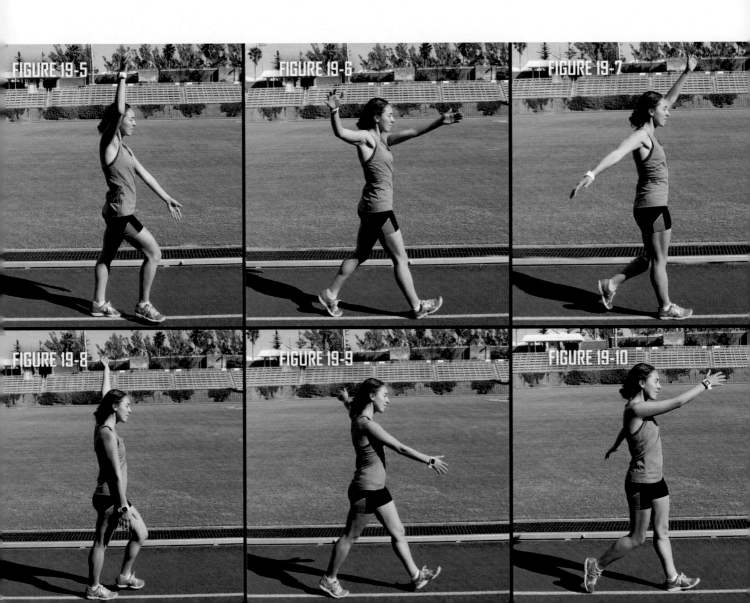

STATIC SHOULDER
STRETCH

A good stretch to add to your cool down is the **_Static Shoulder_** stretch. It helps to relax the shoulders after a walk and increase range of motion.

BODY POSITION

Perform this exercise while standing with your feet approximately a shoulder width apart.

STEPS

A) Attempt to clasp your hands behind your back, one from above and one from below (Figure 19-11); If you can reach, hold the position for 20 to 30 seconds.
B) Reverse arms to stretch the other shoulder.
C) If your hands remain a few inches apart from each other, use a towel or rope to complete the stretch (Figure 19-12).
D) Walk your hands up the rope, positioning them as close together as possible, then reverse arms.

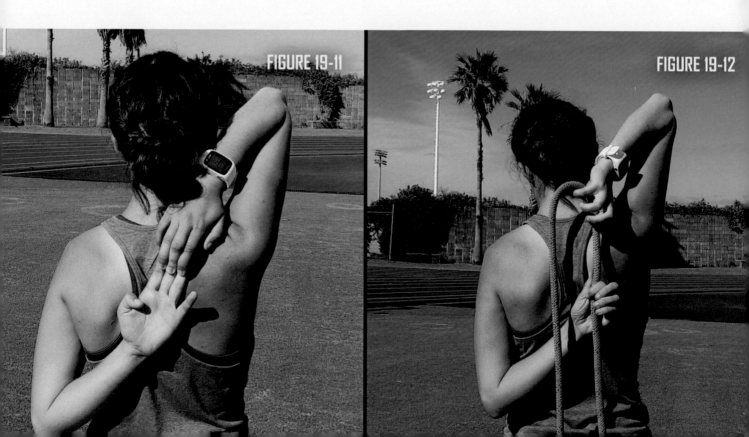

FIGURE 19-11

FIGURE 19-12

NECK STRETCH

Tight neck muscles lead to high shoulders and a higher center of gravity, and thus loss of contact. If only one side is tight, your head could tilt to one side.

BODY POSITION

This stretch can be accomplished from either a seated or standing position.

STEPS

A) Place your palm against the side of your head.
B) Gently push your head to the side so that your ear moves closer to your shoulder (Figure 19-13).
C) Hold for 10-15 seconds.
D) Repeat with the other hand in the opposite direction.

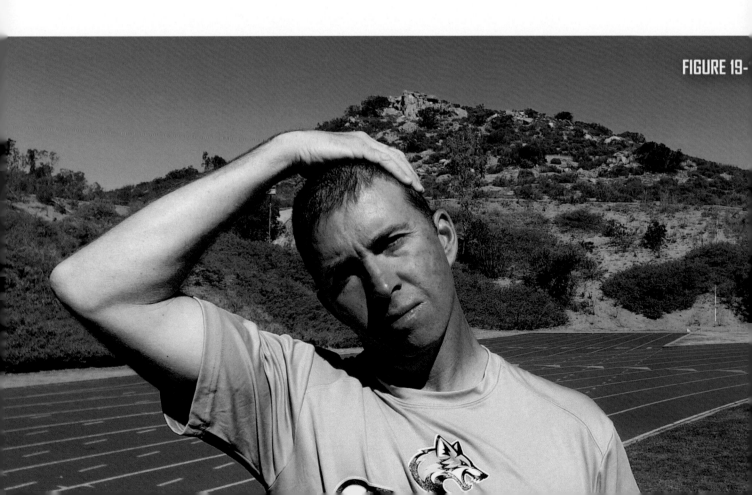

FIGURE 19-

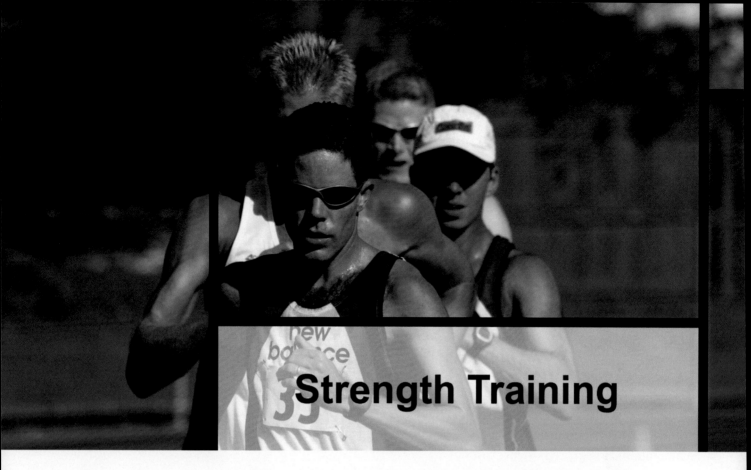

Strength Training

Many endurance athletes believe that lifting heavy weights causes you to bulk up and gain weight. This doesn't have to be the case. The old school philosophy of strength training for endurance athletes used endurance tempo training to combat this. This idea for endurance tempo training turns out not to be ideal of endurance athletes. After all endurance athletes already have endurance training.

It is more beneficial to focus on building strength and power by utilizing a select few full-body exercises. Improving strength and power increases your average power output throughout the race, as well as impacting the "kick" to the finish. Not only can we improve strength and power, these movements help reinforce hip extension that is key to the race walking gait.

To be safe and provide maximum benefits, proper posture and form is vital. When we say proper posture, we mean more than just standing up straight. Proper posture starts with our feet forward, spine and hips in a neutral position, shoulders down and back, and head directly over our spine.

Similar to race walking, where you must maintain proper posture through the race or workout, you must maintain proper posture throughout these exercises. If you perform the exercise improperly, you may be capable of lifting more weight and it may feel easier to complete. Your body gravitates towards incorrect positions, especially as you fatigue. This heightens the risk of injury, so stay focused.

Many people have unique muscular imbalances. Individualized instruction is critical to ensure you are ready to perform the exercises and do them correctly. We cannot stress enough that you seek out a professional to help you with the strength training program introduced here to ensure your posture and form are correct. You may shy away from paying for an experienced trainer, but this investment will really pay off.

Performing exercises incorrectly may allow you to lift more weight and push through more repetitions, but you will be utilizing the wrong muscles and gaining little while risking great personal injury. Please seek assistance, as there are few expenses to race walking training and avoiding injuries will not only make you a better race walker, but save you money in the long run.

Full-body strength training exercises assist you in developing strength and power to help drive you through the race, maximize hip extension, and support or enhance the mechanics of race walking. By increasing your strength, power, and overall athleticism through these lifts, you gain an extra gear and become a more successful race walker and athlete.

These exercises help propel the walker faster by increasing hip extension instead of solely relying on the hip flexors to lift the leg forward!

They strengthen the posterior chain including the hamstrings, glutes, trapezius, and rhomboids, essentially the entire backside. This creates balance in the muscles that push and pull the body while race walking and reduces overuse injuries.

Reducing the number of reps required for endurance training down to two to five repetitions builds power without adding much muscular size. You won't add twenty pounds of muscle on your legs. Using heavy weights with low repetitions increases strength and power of a muscle, while minimizing growth (hypertrophy).

Elite walker Rachel Seaman dramatically increased her strength and power using this approach, while only minimally adding muscular weight to the effect of three pounds. She also significantly reduced her body fat percentage. This is like a fighter who competes in a weight class. He too wants to gain strength and power, but must do this without adding additional size, and becoming disqualified from his weight class.

Strength training is an important aspect to training, but don't plan your training schedule around it. Instead, you should perform your drills and stretches every day. Then plan which days you perform your hard race walking workouts, ideally two per week. Next, schedule your strength training on days other than those of your hard race walking workouts. Like your strenuous race walking days, your strength training days should not be close together. For non-full time athletes, twice a week is sufficient. If you are a full-time athlete like Rachel and Miranda, you might add a third day per week.

It is imperative to learn proper technique for these movements before using weights while performing them. You cannot start off lifting a weight you can only lift two times. Technique needs to be constantly monitored for errors from the beginning as well as when you add weights to the exercises.

Looking at Rachel performing some of these exercises, you would think her form is great. This took a long time to master, just like her race walking technique. Rachel started with a kettlebell instead of a barbell and heavy weight. There were flaws in her posture that impacted her form. You will not see these, but a professional trainer can. She lacked thoracic extension in the spine, and hip capsule mobility restricted her ability to properly perform a deadlift. Had she continued without correcting these issues, she likely would have suffered a severe lumbar spine injury. It took her months of working on form, and postural correction before she got the point where she could pull a 155 pound deadlift with a bodyweight of only 120 pounds. So please, **we can't emphasize enough, if you are going to train with power exercises, seek a professional.**

When lifting weights, the number of repetitions per set fall into three general categories:

* **Power** - 2-5 repetitions which build power without bulk.
* **Strength** - 6-12 repetitions which build strength with bulk.
* **Endurance Lifting** - 20 repetitions which build endurance without bulk

You should start your strength training program at 20 repetitions. How quickly you progress into power repetitions depends on your personal athleticism, ability to learn form, and whether you have any imbalances or postural corrections that must first be addressed.

Before moving into the power phase of 2-5 repetitions, it is important to first spend time building a foundational level of overall strength. This may take months, depending on the individual. Like any training, tapering off prior to competition is important. This includes lowering the number of sets and reps during the week leading up to competition.

2-5
BUILD POWER
NOT BULK
REPS

6-12
BUILD STRENGTH
WITH BULK
REPS

20
BUILD ENDURANCE
NOT BULK
REPS

Miranda and Rachel demonstrate each of the following 12 exercises with light weights for illustrative purposes.

PALLOFF PRESS
EXERCISE

The **Palloff Press** is great for working the core in a way that helps race walking translate core work into functional movement. It also helps train the body for better posture which is critical to the rest of our strength training exercises.

BODY POSITION

- Stand far enough away from the machine or pole so there is some tension in the cable or band.
- Stand with your feet a shoulder width apart, your knees lightly bent, your posture straight up and down, and your pelvis in the neutral position.

STEPS

1. Grab a handle attached to a cable or an elastic band attached to a pole and hold it in line with your sternum (Figure 20-1).
2. Press the cable straight out fully extending your arms; As you do, your core should engage (Figure 20-2).
3. Hold for two seconds and then return your hands to the sternum (Figure 20-1).

Complete your reps and sets from one side and then turn around and face in the opposite direction and repeat.

TAKE CARE!!!

- Do not let the cable pull your body and rotate it towards the machine.
- Resist the temptation to rotate your body from side to side.
- Notice how Miranda keeps her body within the green lines (Figure 20-3).
- Also pay attention to your pelvis.
- It must remain in the neutral position (Figure 20-4).
- Do not tilt your pelvis forward (Figure 20-5) or backward (Figure 20-6).

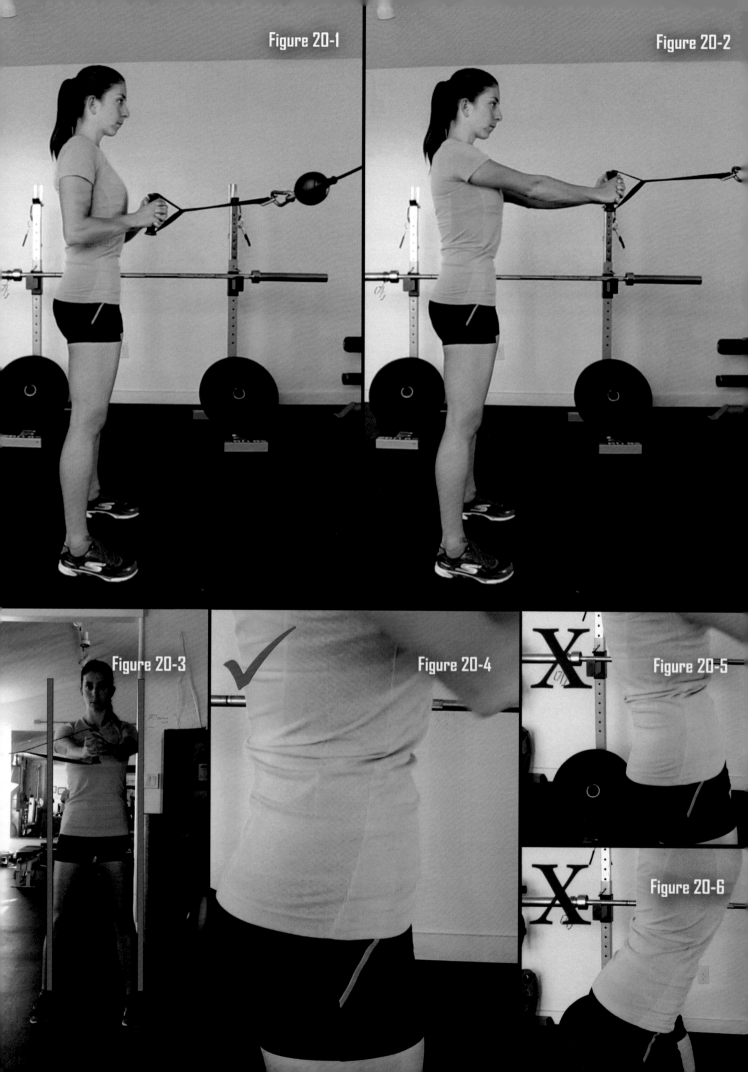

Figure 20-1

Figure 20-2

Figure 20-3

Figure 20-4

Figure 20-5

Figure 20-6

BARBELL DEADLIFT EXERCISE

Barbell Deadlift is one of the best exercises you can do to work your complete posterior chain, aka the muscles along the back of your body. These are the muscles that are largely responsible for forward movement and hip extension.

BODY POSITION

- Place your feet a hip to shoulder width apart and toes pointed slightly outward between 5 to 10 degrees.
- Hold the bar comfortably with your hands more than a shoulder width apart (Figures 20-8 & 20-10)
- The back should be straight at all times.

STEPS

1. Unlock the knees and push the butt backward using your hips as a hinge, the chest falls over the knees as a result with your shoulders in line with the bar.
2. As you go down, bend the knees and they will push out a little, but continue to push the butt backwards (Figure 20-7 & 20-9).
3. Bending from the hips, not the waist, is critical here.
4. It assures the movement is correct and will reduce your chance of injury.

TAKE CARE!!!

- Be careful not to lean back when you reach the top of your lift.
- Pay attention to squeezing the glutes and continuing to keep your back straight as you lift.
- Control the speed as you lower and touch your weights to the floor.
- Although at first you should do this with no weight, as you get more advanced, you can add dumbbells and then progress to a barbell with weights to make the exercise more difficult.

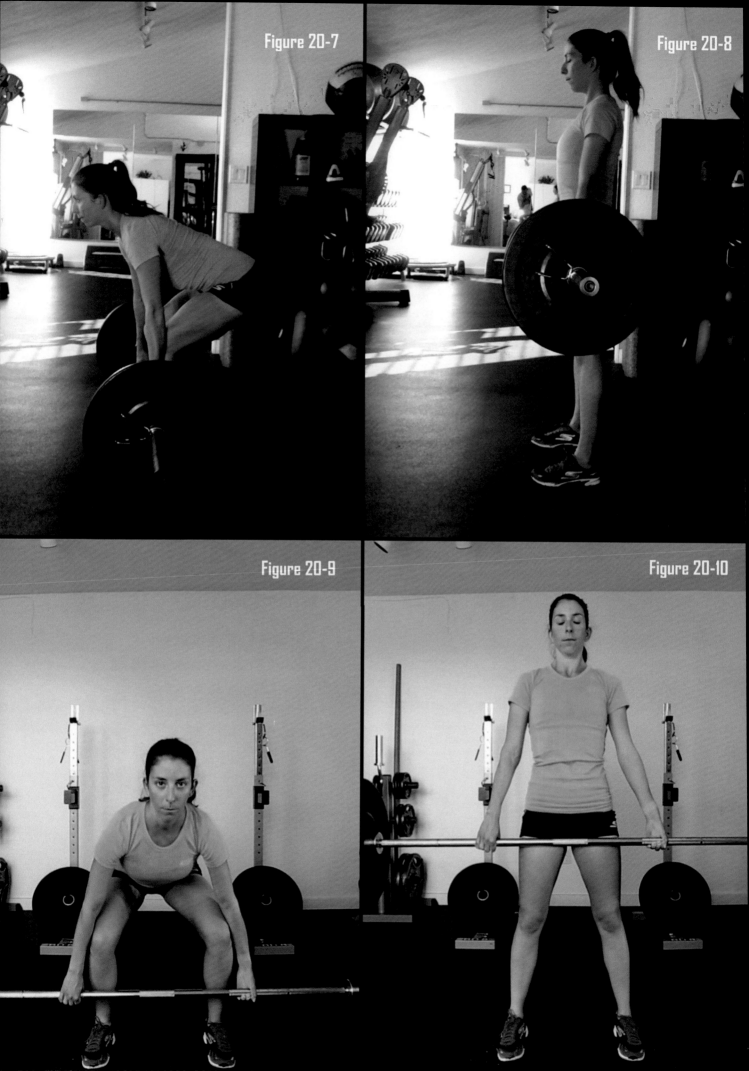

Figure 20-7

Figure 20-8

Figure 20-9

Figure 20-10

BARBELL BACK SQUAT
EXERCISE

The **Barbell Back Squat** is similar to the deadlift in that it's a complete body exercise that focuses on the legs acting on the ankles, knees, and hips. With all joints involved it is a key to top performance and injury prevention for a race walker.

This and the **Barbell Deadlift** are the two exercises that build the most strength and power for a race walker.

BODY POSITION

While your foot position can vary due to personal style, start with your feet at shoulder width apart and pointing forward or a little bit out.

STEPS

1. Place your hands on the bar at about twice the width of your shoulders.
2. Lift the bar behind your head, while keeping your wrists straight, rest the bar on your shoulders, not your spine (Figure 20-12 & 20-14).
3. Bend from the hips, not the waist, as it assures the movement is correct and will reduce your chance of injury; The back should be straight at all times.
4. Lower the body and bar until your upper legs are parallel with the floor (Figures 20-11 & 20-13).
5. Sit back, like you are sitting in a chair and then return to the upright position.

TAKE CARE!!!

- Do not lower your torso below your knees.
- Make sure that your heels are always on the ground and the body's weight is over them.
- Keep your wrists straight throughout.
- Although at first you should do this with no weight, as you get more advanced, you can add dumbbells and then progress to a barbell with weights to make the exercise more difficult.

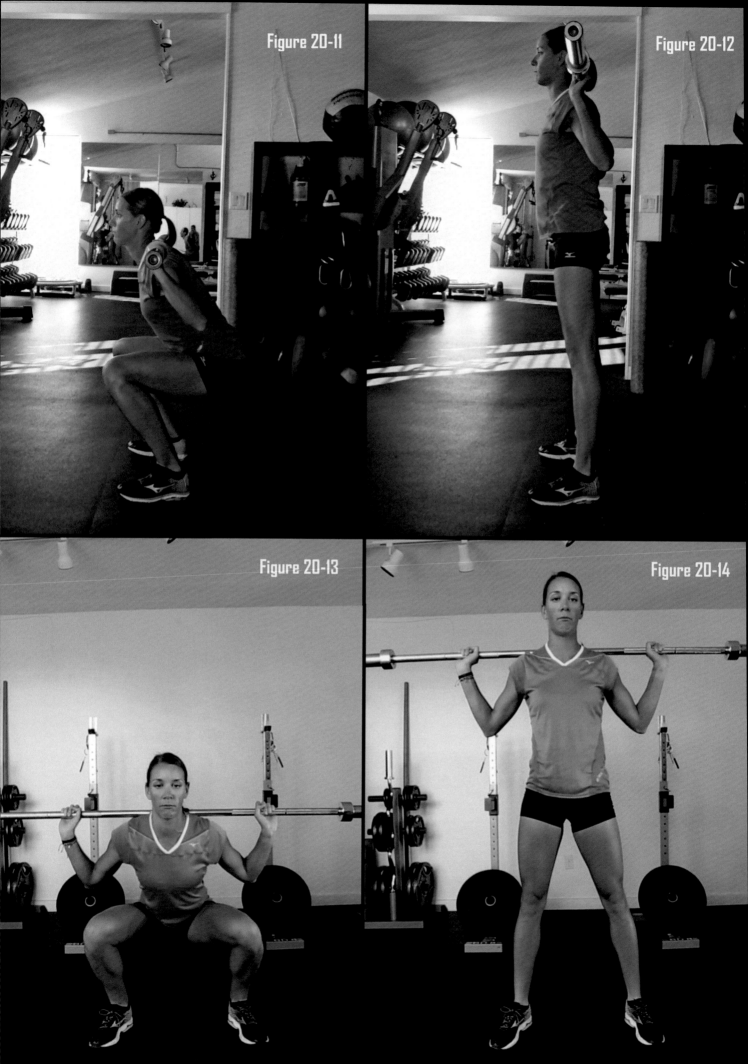

Figure 20-11

Figure 20-12

Figure 20-13

Figure 20-14

BULGARIAN SPLIT SQUAT
EXERCISE

Much like the **Barbell Back Squat**, the **Bulgarian Split Squat** works the hip, knee and ankle joints, however, being a single leg exercise, it brings in joint stability similar to the needs of a race walker at heel strike.

BODY POSITION

Stand with your front foot on the ground, with the knee directly above the ankle and your back foot on a bench or chair (Figures 20-16 & 20-18).

STEPS

1. Lower your body by bending the front knee to a 90 degree angle (Figures 20-15 & 20-17).
2. Keep your upper body upright with a neutral pelvis throughout the entire movement.

TAKE CARE!!!

Beginners should do this with no weight, but as you get more advanced, you can add dumbbells or a medicine ball to make the exercise more difficult.

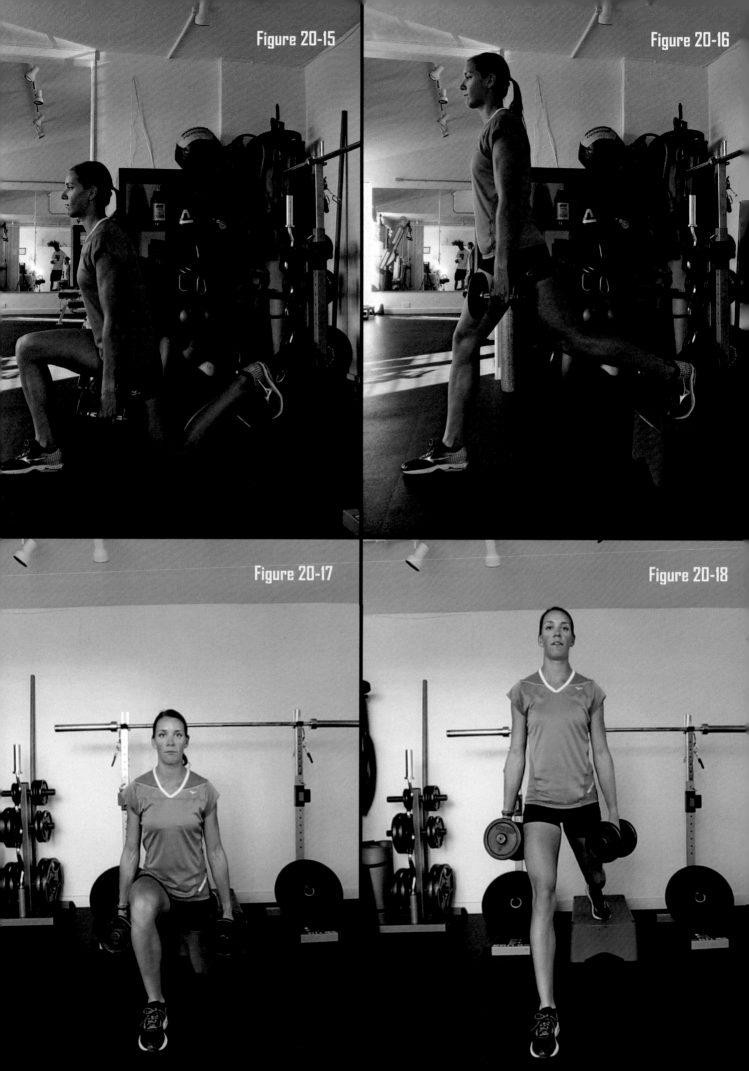

Figure 20-15

Figure 20-16

Figure 20-17

Figure 20-18

SINGLE LEG DEADLIFTS
EXERCISE

The **Single Leg Deadlift** is like the **Barbell Deadlift** in that this exercise emphasizes the posterior chain. However, being a single leg exercise, it brings in joint stability similar to the needs of a race walker at heel strike. This is a more advanced version of the deadlift accomplished with a single supporting leg that develops the hamstrings.

BODY POSITION

Stand with your weight on a slightly bent leg (Figures 20-20 & 20-22).

STEPS

1. Bend forward at the hips, not the waist, keeping your back straight throughout the exercise.
2. As you lean forward your free leg raises and is kept mostly straight.
3. Continue leaning forward until the body and free leg are close to parallel with the ground (Figures 20-19 & 20-21). Pause for a second in this position and return to the standing position.

TAKE CARE!!!

- You may want a chair, bench or stationary pole available in front of you for balance.
- Beginners should do this with no weight. As you get more advanced, you can add dumbbells.

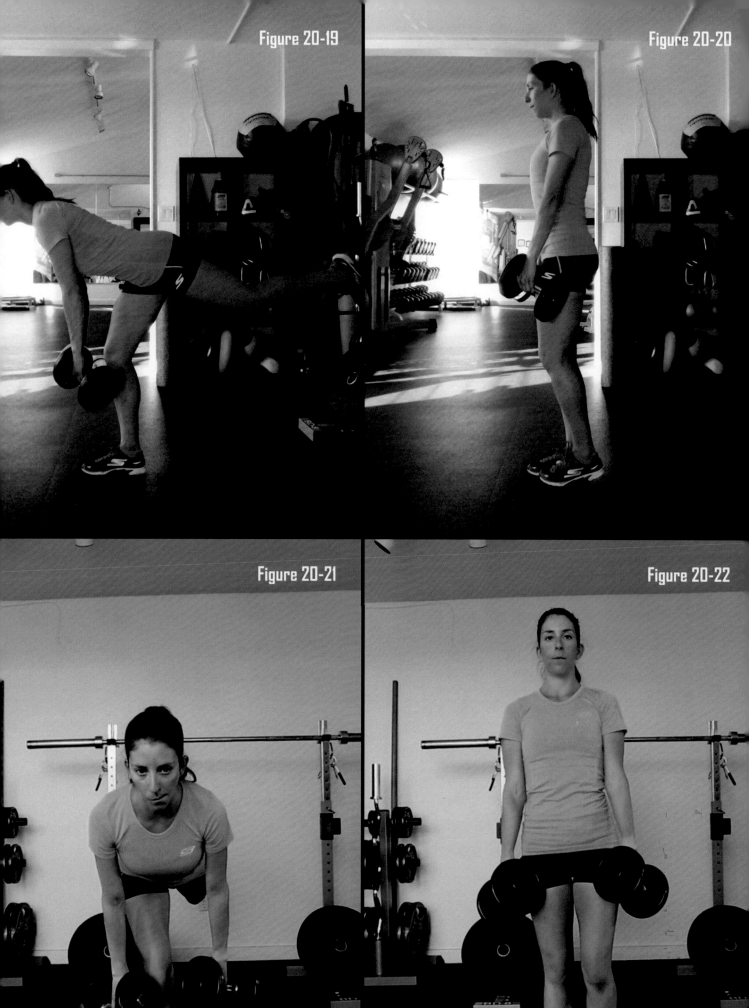

Figure 20-19

Figure 20-20

Figure 20-21

Figure 20-22

DOUBLE DUMBBELL STEP UPS
EXERCISE

The **Double Dumbbell Step Up** is similar to a **Bulgarian Split Squat** from a pattern standpoint, requiring the ankles, knees, and hips to go through full ranges of motions. However, it brings the challenge of joint stability because it is performed on a single leg. This is crucial to the race walker.

BODY POSITION

The **Double Dumbbell Step Up** can be performed on a step, chair, bench, or other secure platform at varying heights.

STEPS

1. Step up onto the platform and raise your body up so that your support leg is fully straightened (Figures 20-24 & 20-26).
2. You then lower yourself back down to the ground (Figures 20-23 & 20-25).
3. Repeat this with the same leg for as many repetitions as you want to perform for the set and then switch legs.

TAKE CARE!!!

- Beginners should do this with no weight.
- As you get more advanced, you can add dumbbells.

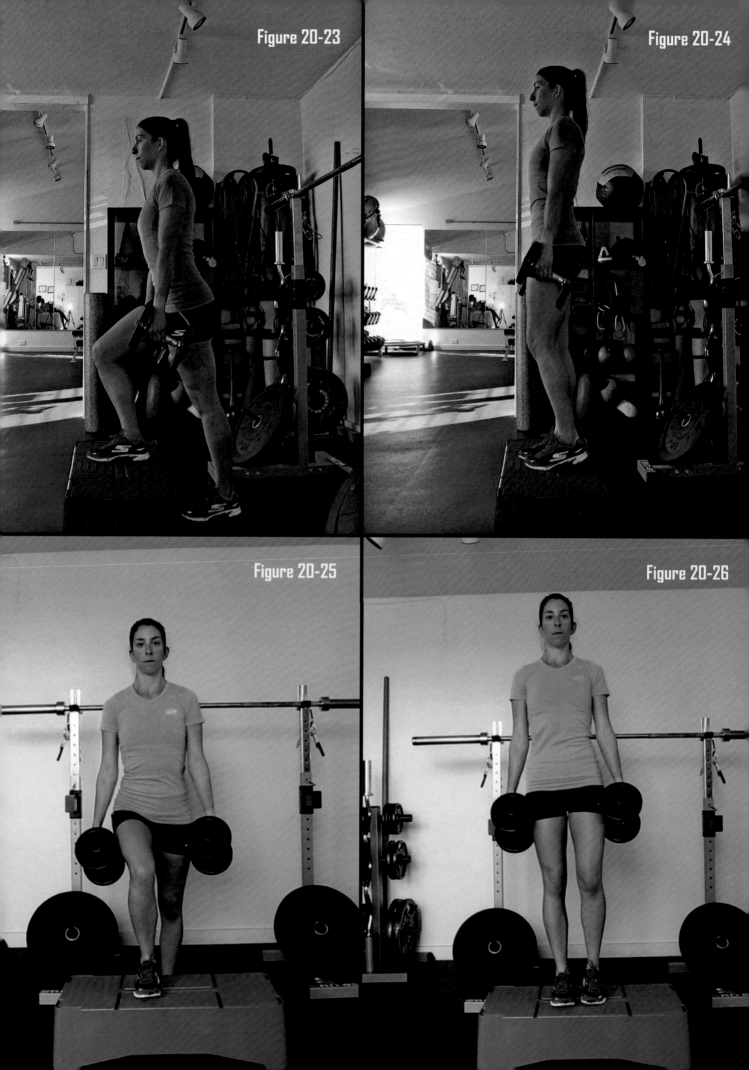

Figure 20-23

Figure 20-24

Figure 20-25

Figure 20-26

KETTLEBELL SWING
EXERCISE

The **Kettlebell Swing** is the **Hip Hinge** or top portion of the **Deadlift**. However, it is done explosively to develop power.

BODY POSITION

Stand with your feet slightly more than shoulder width apart and keep your elbows locked.

STEPS

1. Grasp the kettle bell with an overhand grip with both hands.
2. Start by swinging the kettlebell backward through your legs to gain some momentum like the downward movement of the squat (Figures 20-27 & 20-29).
3. Then, drive the kettlebell upward from your hips, as you stand up, raising the weight to a maximum height of the shoulder (Figures 20-28 & 20-39), while forming two straight lines. One through your back and the other through your arms.
4. As you lower the bell, let gravity be your friend, and allow it to lower the bell.

TAKE CARE!!!

- Be careful when finishing not to just stop the motion in mid swing. Allow the kettlebell to lower and carefully place it on the ground.
- **This exercise requires you to have mastered the *Deadlift* as it is central in its execution.**

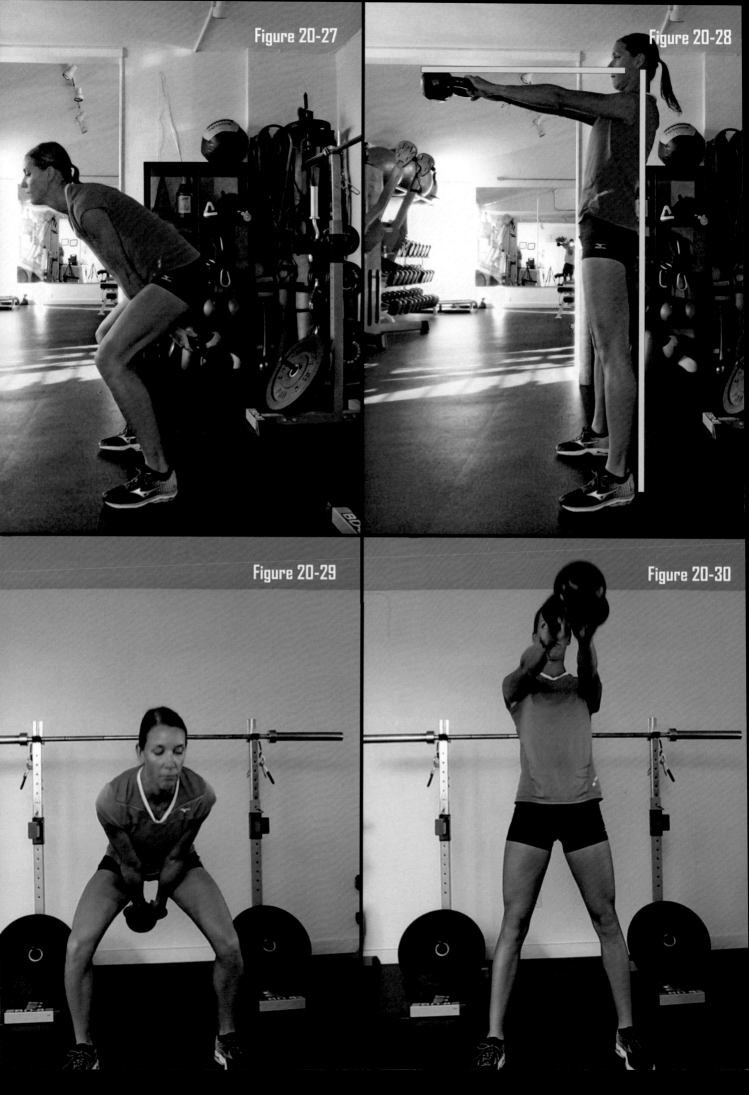

Figure 20-27

Figure 20-28

Figure 20-29

Figure 20-30

DUMBBELL WALKING LUNGE
EXERCISE

Dumbbell Walking Lunge is a more advanced version of a **Split Squat**, adding movement that increases the demands on your joint stability.

BODY POSITION

Start from a normal standing position.

STEPS

1. Step forward with one leg (Figure 20-31), landing on the heel, not on the forefoot.
2. Once you are in this straddling position, while keeping your body upright, bend the front leg at the knee (Figure 20-32).
3. Then lower your body at the hips until the back knee almost touches the ground (Figure 20-33).
4. It is important that your forward step is far enough that the knee stays over the ankle and does not push over the toes.
5. Then begin to stand back up and repeat these actions on the other leg.

TAKE CARE!!!

*   Mastering these movements is critical before trying to add weights to them.
*   Some may even wish to start with a standing lunge exercise before moving on to the walking exercise.

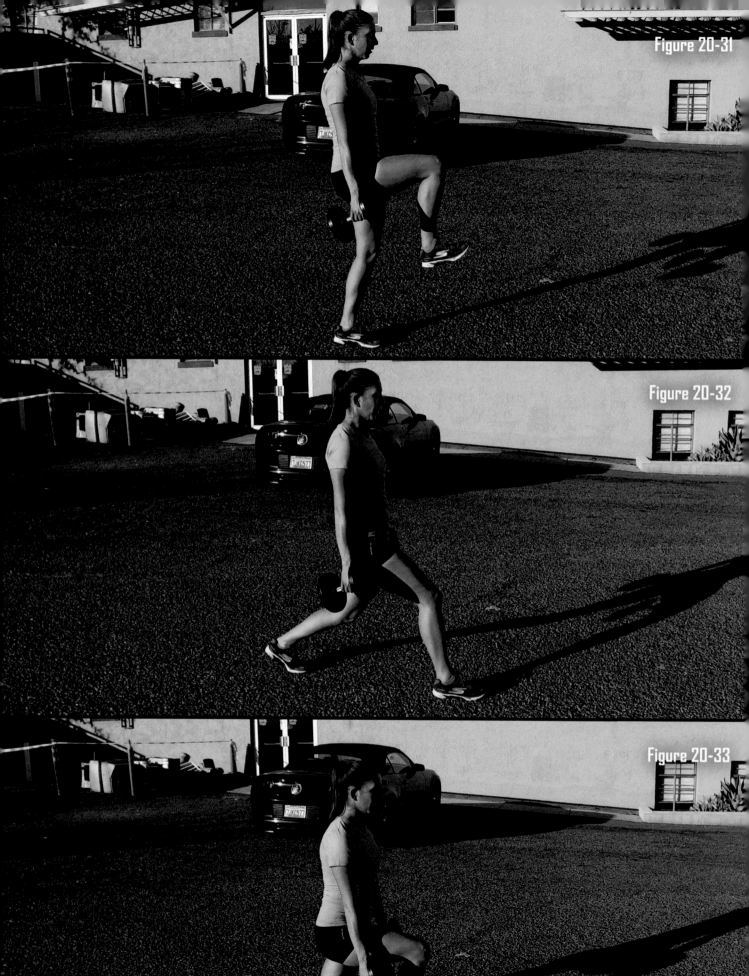

Figure 20-31

Figure 20-32

Figure 20-33

CABLE CHOP
EXERCISE

The **Cable Chop** is an advanced version of the **Palloff Press** with an added rotation that increases the workload of your core to stabilize your neutral position and maintain your proper race walking posture.

BODY POSITION

Stand with your feet slightly more than a shoulder width apart.

STEPS

1. Grab the handle of the cable at chest height (Figures 20-34 & 20-36).
2. Start with the weight on your inside leg and while keeping the back straight rotate outward pulling the cable across your body in a horizontal movement. As you do, pivot on your inside foot and shift the weight to your outside foot. Allow your head to track with your body so you are constantly looking at your hands (Figures 20-35 & 20-37).
3. Repeat this on one side for as many repetitions as you want to perform for the set and then switch sides.

TAKE CARE!!!

- Your torso and arms do the movement, but be careful not to lead your motion by leaning into the direction you are rotating,
- Be careful not to swing all the way back.

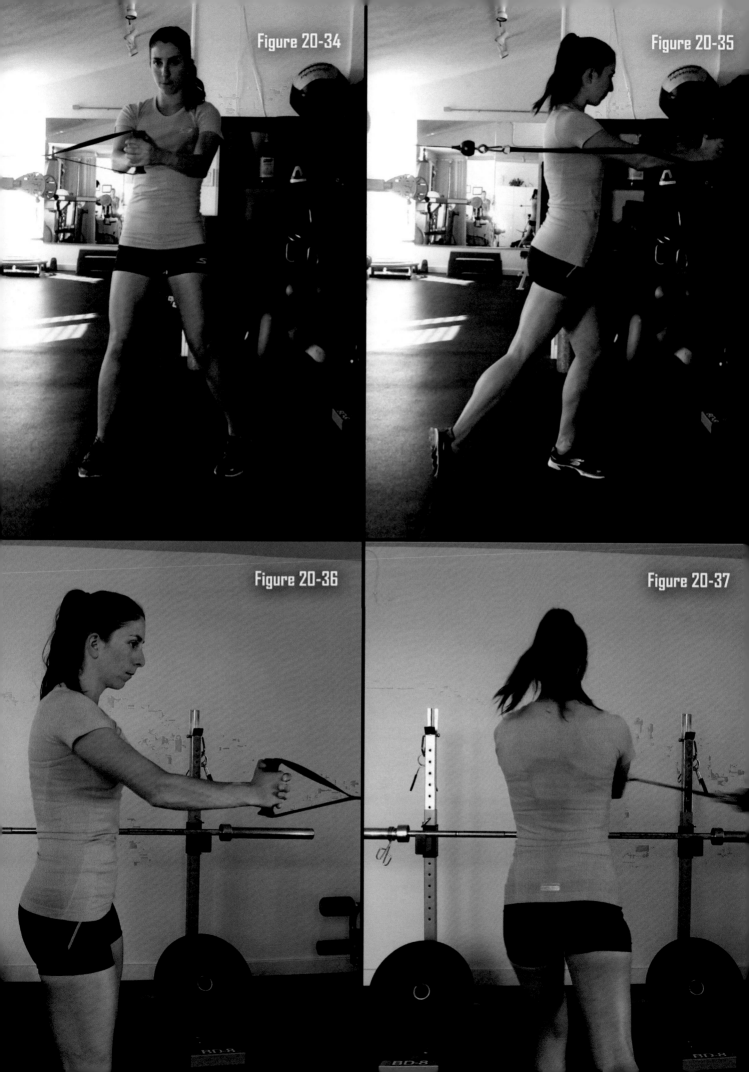

Figure 20-34

Figure 20-35

Figure 20-36

Figure 20-37

CABLE PUNCH
EXERCISE

The **Cable Punch** is a core stability exercise that integrates a neutral spine and pelvis while forcing you to stabilize the core as well as the ankles, knees, and hips. This teaches your core to turn on while maintaining a neutral pelvis, which translates well to race walking.

BODY POSITION

Stand with your feet shoulder width apart.

STEPS

1. Grab the handle of the cable at shoulder height with the hand closer to the machine.
2. Start with the leg closer to the machine behind you and your other leg in front of you (Figures 20-38 & 20-40).
3. Simultaneously step forward with the rear leg and punch forward with your corresponding arm. At the end of the punch your arms should be fully extended (Figures 20-39 & 20-41).
4. Step backwards with the corresponding arm retreating as well (Figures 20-38 & 20-40).
5. Repeat this on one side for as many repetitions as you want to perform for the set and then switch sides.

TAKE CARE!!!

Take care to maintain a straight back and neutral pelvis throughout the exercise.

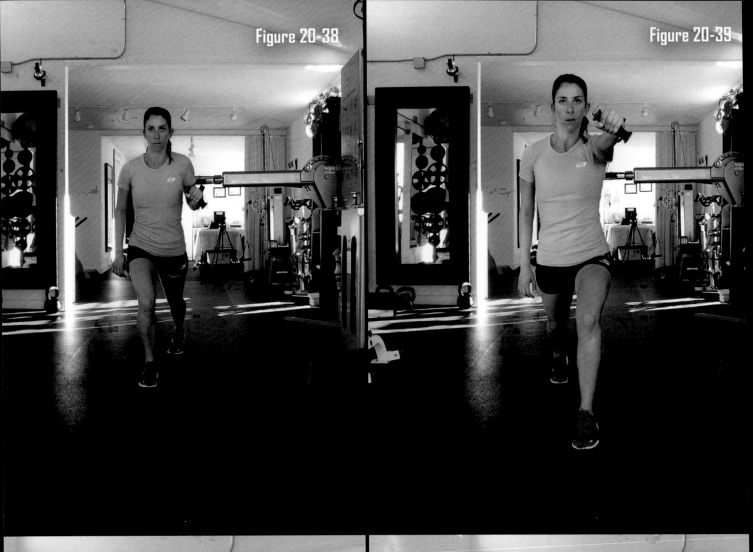

Figure 20-38

Figure 20-39

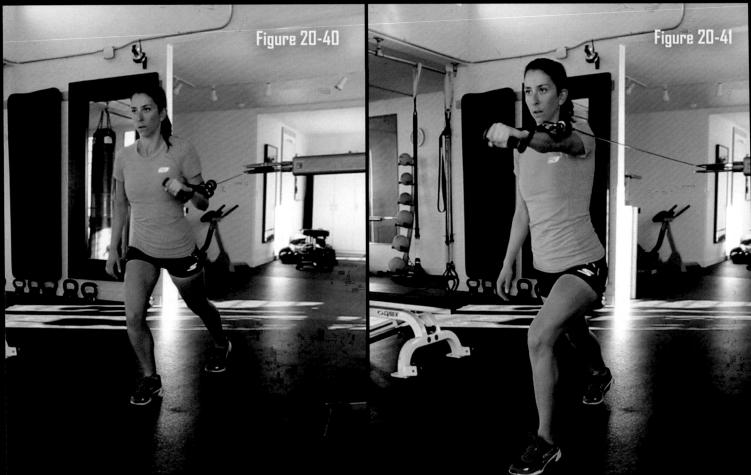

Figure 20-40

Figure 20-41

TURKISH GET UP 1

EXERCISE

The **Turkish Get Up 1** is a core exercise that does not activate the hip flexors and forces you into thoracic extension which helps correct a common rounded shoulder posture that many endurance athletes suffer from.

BODY POSITION

Lie on the floor and straighten your right leg while keeping your left leg knee bent at a 90 degree angle.

STEPS

1. Hold your straightened left arm up, keeping your back against the floor (Figure 20-42).
2. Reach up for the ceiling, rotating your torso and using your right arm, bent at about 90 degrees, to help support your weight (Figure 20-43).
3. Slowly lower your torso and arm, but keep the arm up and straightened (Figure 20-42).
4. Repeat this on one side for as many repetitions as you want to perform for the set and then switch sides.

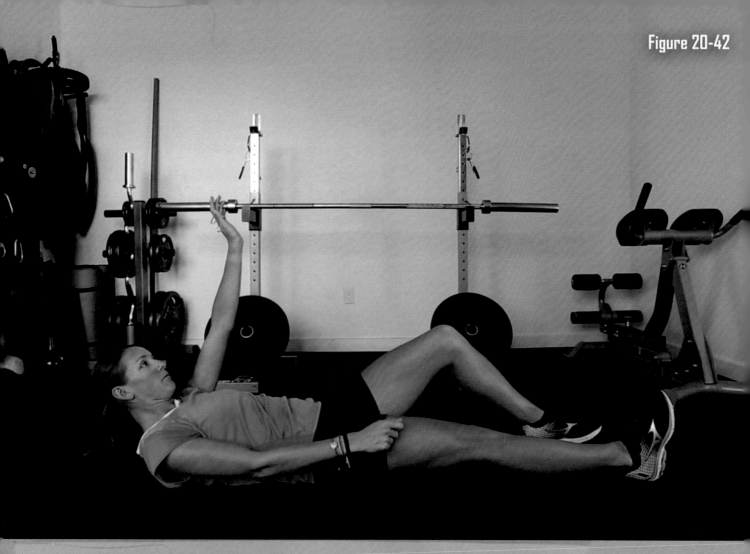

Figure 20-42

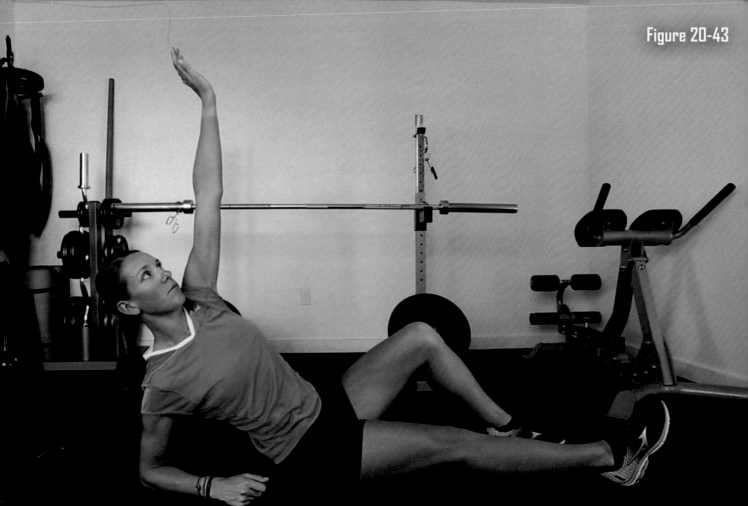

Figure 20-43

RACE WALKERS IN MOTION

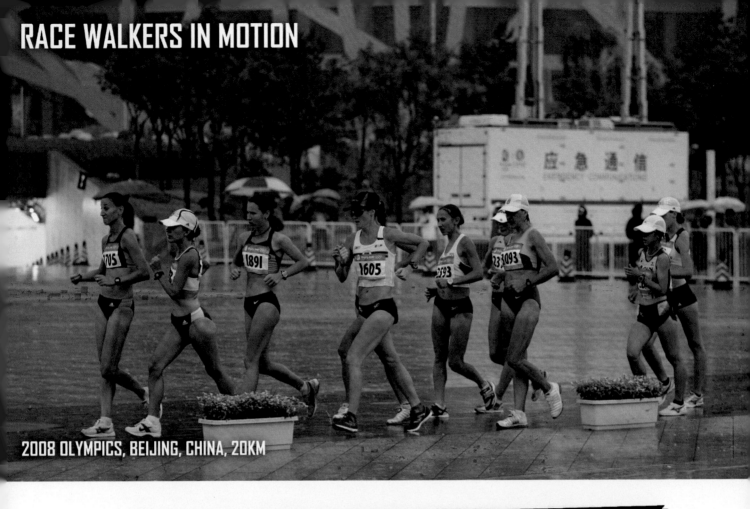

2008 OLYMPICS, BEIJING, CHINA, 20KM

TURKISH GET UP 2
EXERCISE

The *Turkish Get Up 2* is a variation on the previous *Turkish Get Up 1*.

BODY POSITION

Lay on the ground with both legs extended, keep the knees slightly bent and hold your arms so they are perpendicular to the ground (Figure 20-44).

STEPS

1. With both arms extended sit up reaching for the ceiling until your torso is in the vertical position and your arms are directly in line with your torso (Figure 20-45).
2. Slowly return to the floor and repeat.

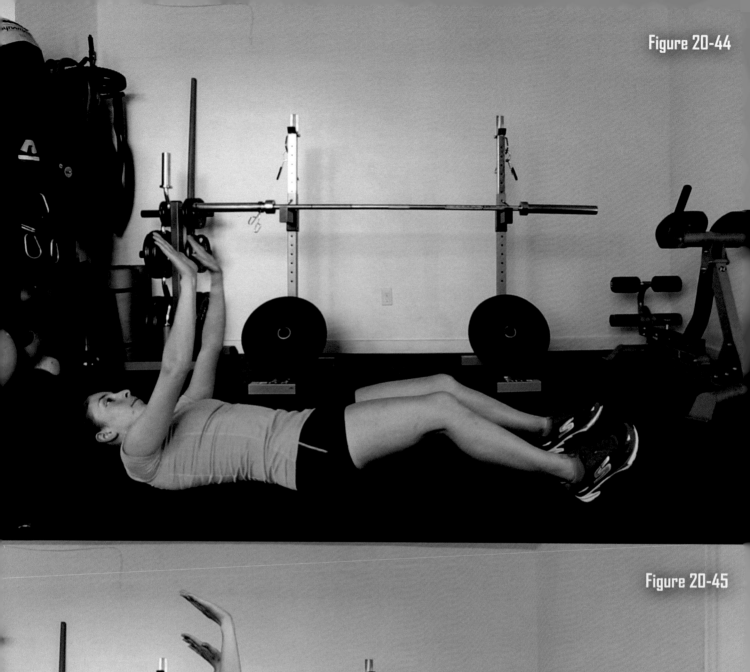

Figure 20-44

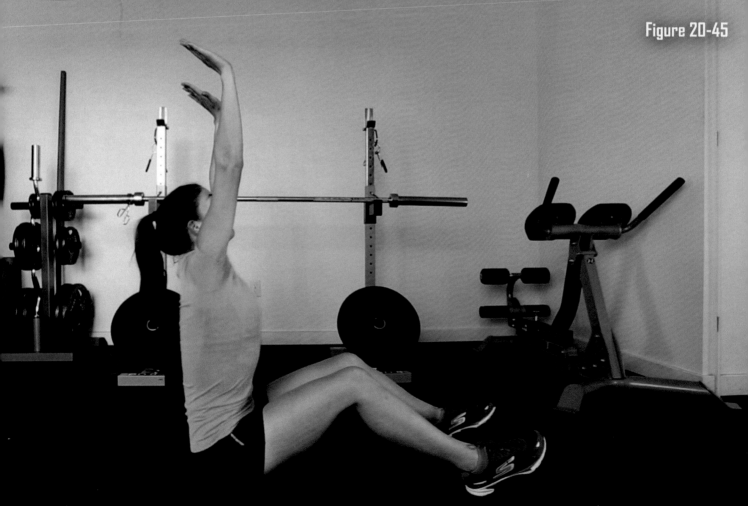

Figure 20-45

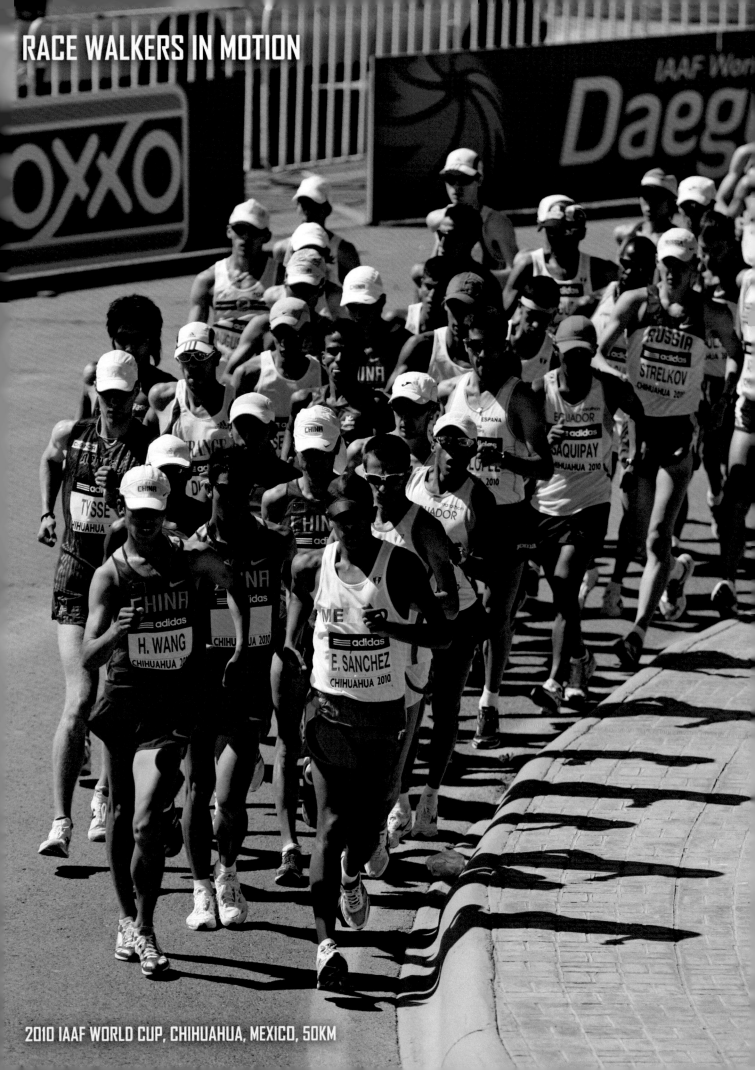

RACE WALKERS IN MOTION

2010 IAAF WORLD CUP, CHIHUAHUA, MEXICO, 50KM

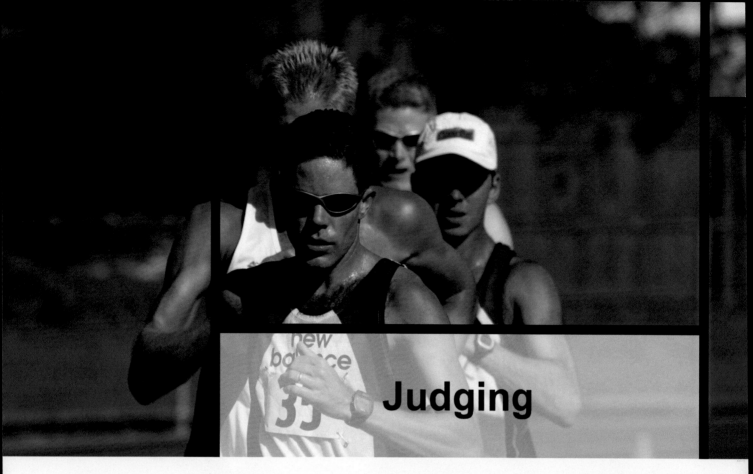

Judging

An entire book can be written about how to judge race walking. However, as an athlete you should know the best practices a judge follows while observing you. If you see a judge violating these practices, it is best not to call them out during the race, but you might politely discuss it with them afterward.

A race walking judge evaluates a competitive race walker for legality based on two parts of the race walking definition: loss of contact and bent knee.

When determining whether a walker hasn't maintained contact with the ground, a judge should only look at the walker's feet and not be influenced by the hands, head, knees or other parts of the body.

A judge also looks to see that a walker's advancing leg appears straightened from the moment of first contact with the ground until in the vertical position.

A judge should not determine the legality of a race walker from the front or behind (Figure 21-1). Instead a judge should observe the walkers when the athletes approach the judge's field of view from 45 degrees as they advance towards the judge through 15 degrees past the judge (Figure 21-2).

However, angle alone is not enough, when a judge stands too close to the walkers it's very difficult to get an accurate view of their technique. Instead, a judge should stand 20 to 30 feet away from approaching walkers. It is very difficult to judge the legality of a race walker when you

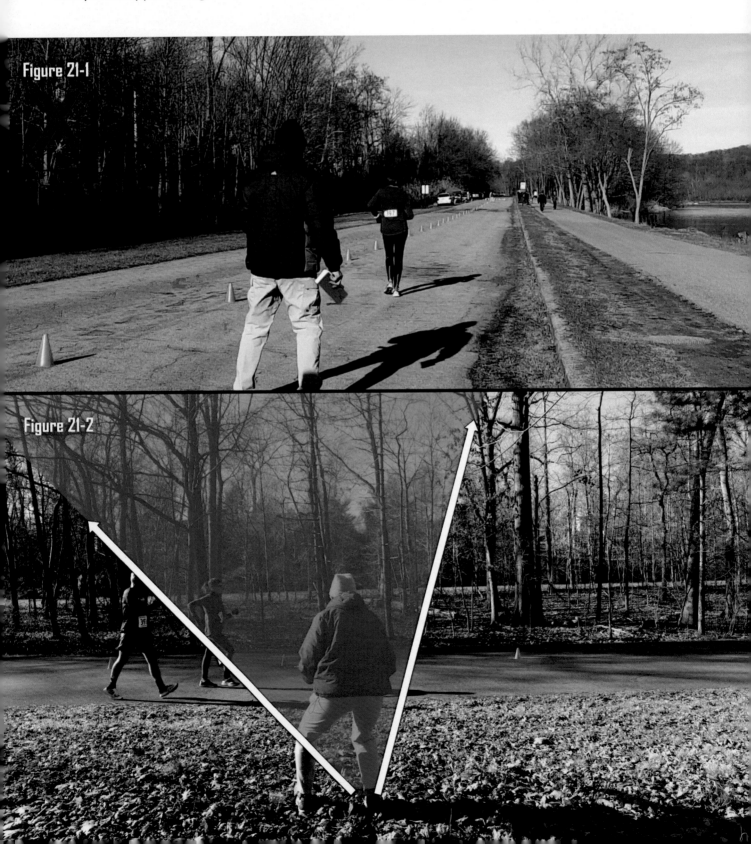

Figure 21-1

Figure 21-2

stand only 5 feet away (Figure 21-3). If you judge from the proper angle, but not the proper distance, that gives you less than 4 steps to determine legality. The situation is even more difficult if you have more than one walker racing by (Figure 21-4). From 10 feet away, you have 5-6 steps to judge (Figure 21-5). In contrast, when you judge from at least 20 feet away, you have 10 steps to determine legality (Figure 21-6).

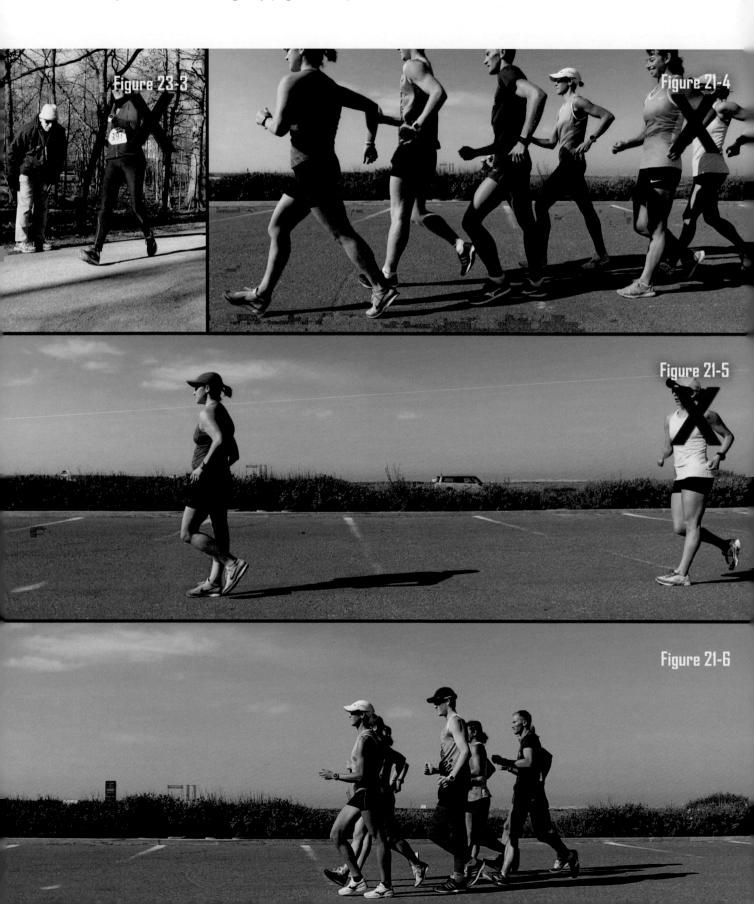

Figure 23-3

Figure 21-4

Figure 21-5

Figure 21-6

Judges should also never follow a walker as they go by (Figure 21-7). Judges act independently of each other and should not communicate their findings during the event (Figure 21-8). A judge should never need to crawl on the ground or hide behind a tree or other obstacle (Figure 21-9).

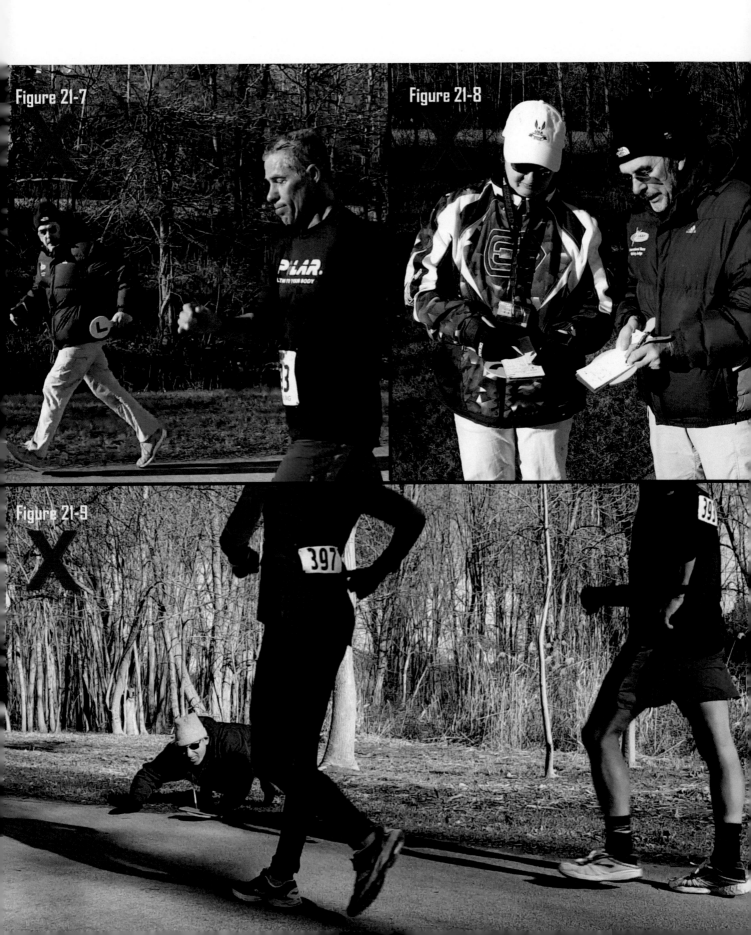

Figure 21-7

Figure 21-8

Figure 21-9

If a judge believes you are in danger of violating either portion of the definition of race walking, a judge should show you a yellow paddle with the proper symbol for the potential violation: loss of contact (Figure 21-10) or bent-knee (Figure 21-11).

A judge may only show you a yellow paddle once for each type of infraction. If, however, a judge believes you are in violation of the definition of race walking, they submit a red card which is a proposal for disqualification. A judge may only submit one proposal for disqualification per race walker. They do not inform the athlete of this action. Instead, the athlete sees a dot or symbol next to their race number on a red card posting board similar to the one shown in Figure 21-13. Additionally, an athlete may usually request to see the judges' summary sheet after the race.

In the simplest case, it takes three proposals for disqualification from three different judges to be disqualified. In some races, a pit lane is employed, and then a fourth proposal for disqualification is required. Also, during certain international competitions and USATF national championships, the chief judge may disqualify a race walker with only one call during the last 100 meters of the race if the race walker if flagrantly breaking the definition of race walking. A chief judge shows a walker the red paddle (Figure 21-12) to inform a walker that they have been disqualified from the race. The race walker must leave the course.

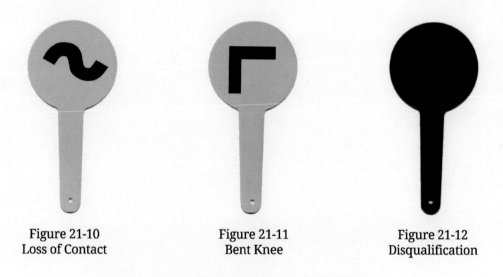

Figure 21-10
Loss of Contact

Figure 21-11
Bent Knee

Figure 21-12
Disqualification

1009	1366 X	1578
1050	1389 X	1606
1056	1415	1894
1185	1504 XX	2019 XX
1201	1543	2070 X
1203 X	1544 X	2131 XXX
1228	1548 X	2161
1346	1574	2178 X

Figure 21-13

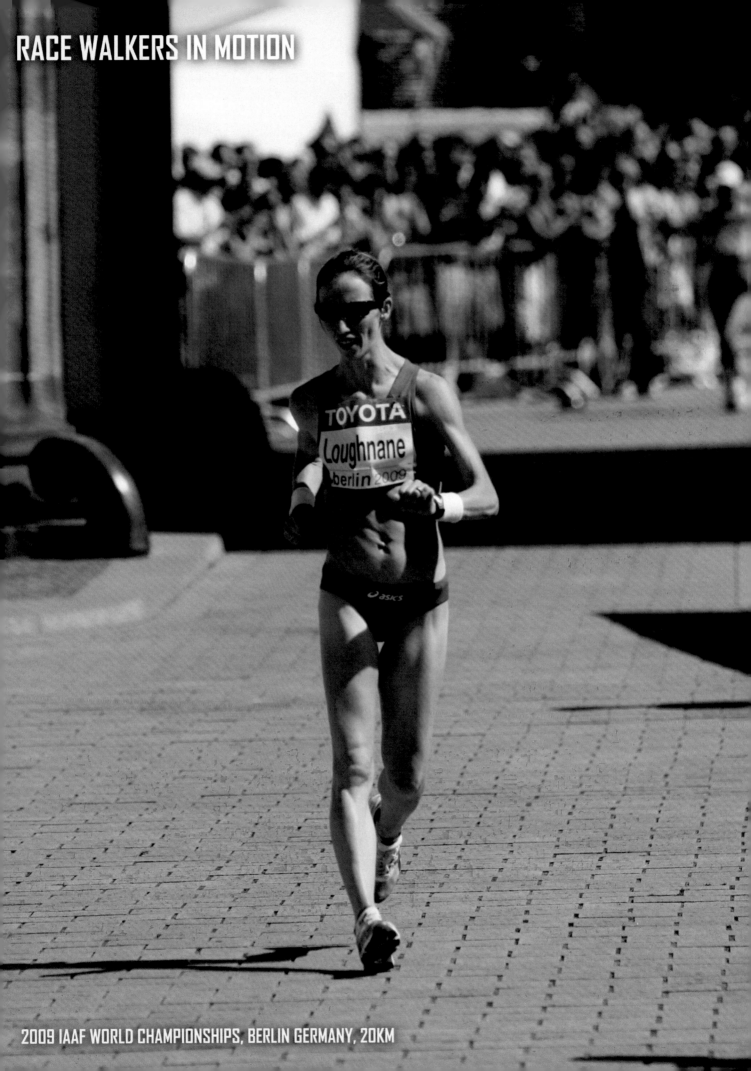

RACE WALKERS IN MOTION

2009 IAAF WORLD CHAMPIONSHIPS, BERLIN GERMANY, 20KM

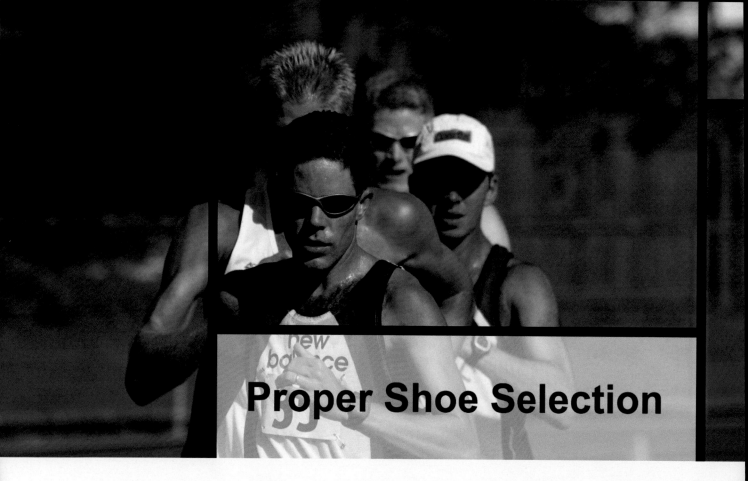

Proper Shoe Selection

Race walking has a blessing and a curse in that the only equipment you need is a good pair of shoes that fit well. The problem is, at any given time there are few, if any, athletic shoes specifically designed for race walkers.

Look at a walker's closet and you'll find a littered mess of shoes. Some are severely worn out and hung onto because their beloved model was discontinued. While others are in pristine condition, because they just weren't right for race walking. The search for the perfect shoe is an ongoing challenge for race walkers. The answer is simple in theory, but difficult to implement.

Most race walkers resort to finding a pair of running shoes, usually long distance racing flats, that have the following characteristics.

A Low Heel

Race walkers strike the ground with significantly less impact and therefore do not need the level of cushioning found in most traditional running shoes. Observe the difference between the heels of a shoe specifically designed for race walking with a support-focused running shoe (Figure 22-1).

However, care must be taken when selecting a shoe with a low heel. If the heel is too cushiony, it might collapse under heel strike as shown with the shoes in Figure 22-3. Even the shoe in Figure 22-2 compresses more than desirable, although it is not as bad as the shoe in Figure 22-3.

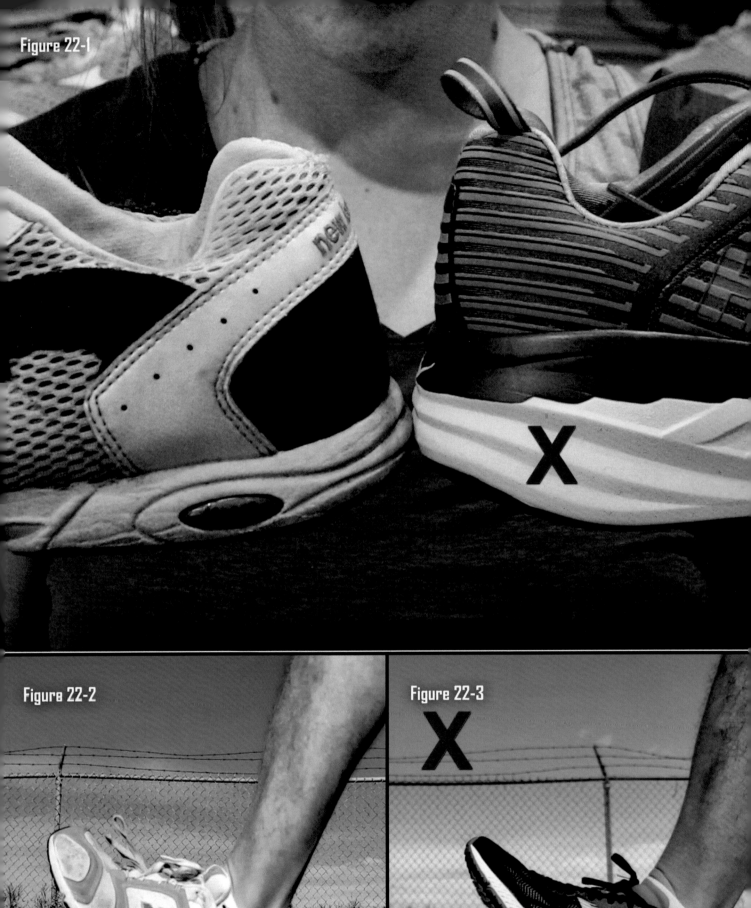

Figure 22-1

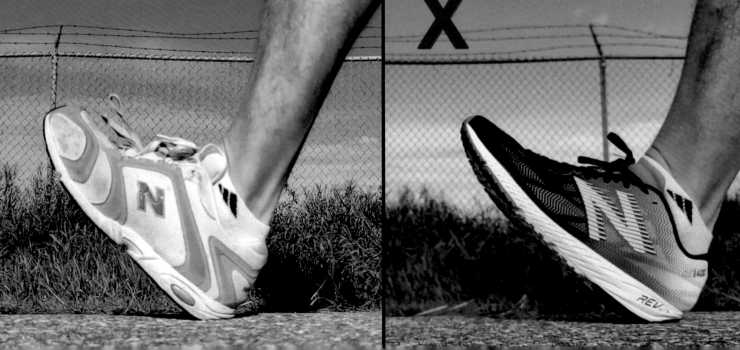

Figure 22-2

Figure 22-3

Proper Flex in the Sole

The sole of the shoe should flex in the right places, but not the wrong places. Flexibility under the ball of the foot (Figure 22-4) is desirable to facilitate a stronger push off behind the body. A lack of rigidity under the arch of the shoe is bad. It leads to the shoe collapsing under the middle of the weight-bearing foot (Figure 22-5), causing the hamstring muscle to elongate in a manner that leads to injuries.

Ample Toe Box

The toe box must have enough room for the foot to spread out comfortably (Figure 22-6). This reduces the chances of injuries like black toe nails. It also facilitates a more substantial push off.

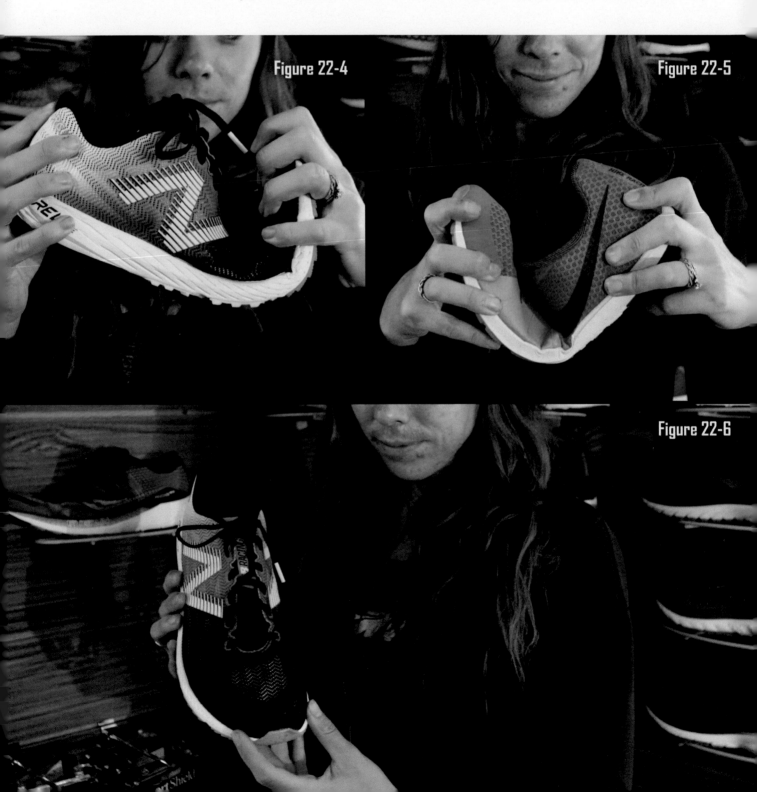

Figure 22-4

Figure 22-5

Figure 22-6

Sturdy Heel Counter

A sturdy heel counter or heel cup is desirable but may be the hardest characteristic to find in a running shoe. With more support in the heel, a race walker gets more rigidity where they need it at heel strike (Figure 22-7).

Be wary of shoes where the heel simply collapses under pressure (Figure 22-8).

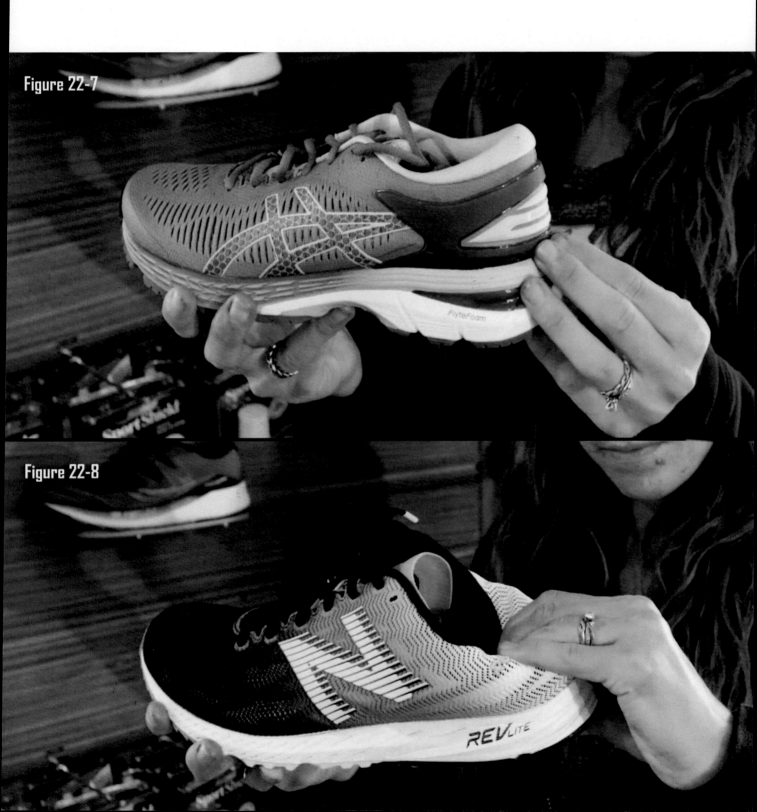

Figure 22-7

Figure 22-8

The Proper Last

When a walker's foot strikes the ground, it lands on the outer corner of the heel (Figure 22-9). As the stride progresses, the foot rolls towards the big toe. The degree that the foot rolls inward indicates the degree of pronation in a walker's stride.

Walkers with an overly inward pronation require a straight-lasted shoe.

Walkers without enough inward pronation, those who supinate or under-pronate, require a curve-lasted shoe.

If you are fortunate enough to pronate normally, then select a semi-curved last.

However, selecting a shoe with the proper last (Figure 22-10) can be difficult. It's best to ask a professional for help.

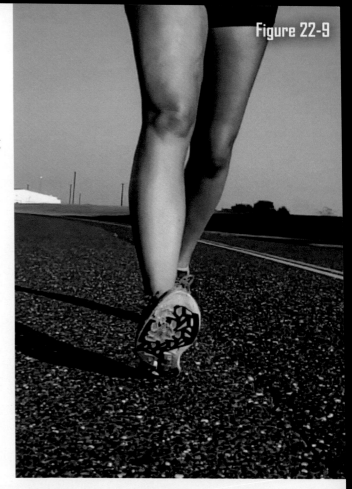

Figure 22-9

Additionally, the rear of the shoe needs to provide **enough room for your Achilles** tendon and thus it should have a notch in the back as shown (Figure 22-11).

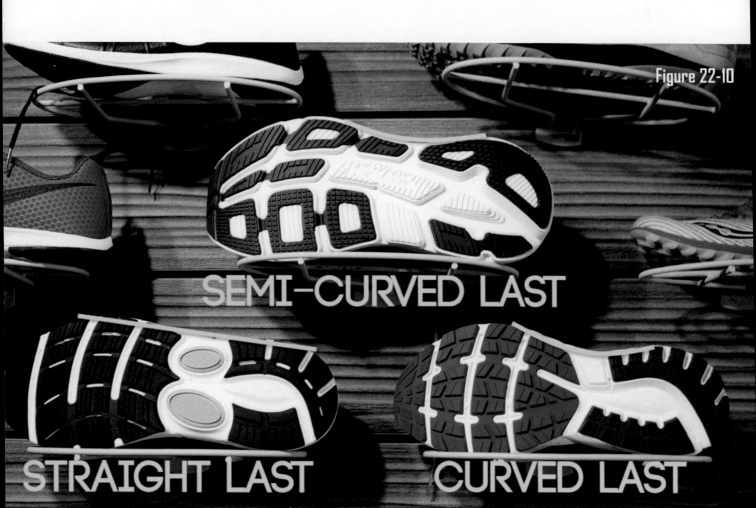

Figure 22-10

SEMI-CURVED LAST

STRAIGHT LAST

CURVED LAST

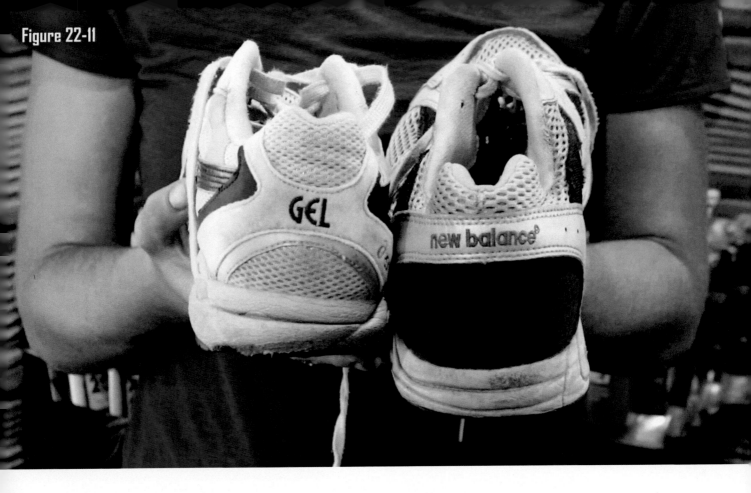

Figure 22-11

Where to Buy

So how can you decide on what shoe is right? We recommend going to store that:

- specializes in running shoes
- are operated by athletically-minded individuals
- who can watch how your walk / run and determine the best shoes for you.

You should know that all running stores won't be familiar with the needs of a race walker, but if you bring them this list of characteristics, they can match your specific needs with these features, fit you properly and ensure you have the best selection available.

Replacing Shoes

A final note, don't wear your shoes too long. Everyone is different. Observe shoes from Olympians Tim Seaman and Miranda Melville (Figure 22-12). Both are excessively worn. When shoes have holes and worn out tread, it's clear that they should be replaced. However, shoes may need to be replaced sooner, if the shoe warps to one side or is unevenly compressed it's time for them to go. Remember, the cost of new shoes is trivial in comparison to the cost of an injury.

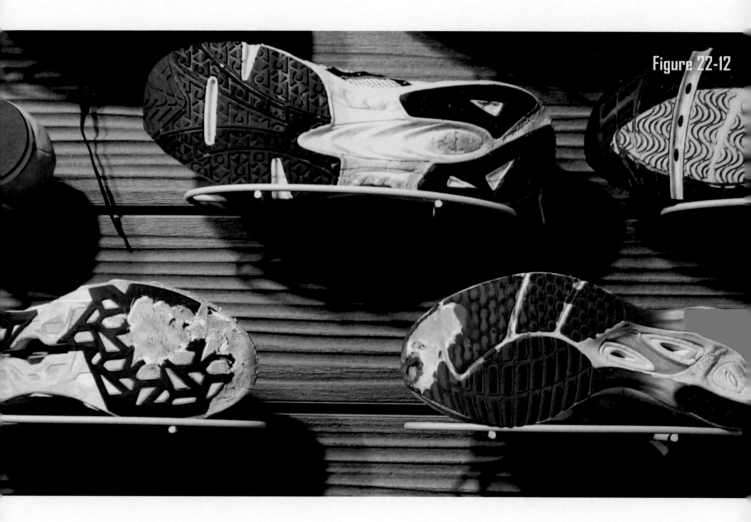

Figure 22-12

Epilogue

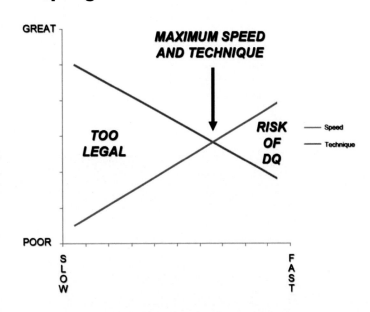

We end *Race Walking Revolution* with a simple graph that illustrates how to balance speed with technique. If you walk too fast, your technique suffers and your risk of disqualification is high. On the contrary, if you focus too much on textbook technique, you speed naturally slows and your performance suffers. It's all about balance. Balance your training, technique work, and remedial drills and your performances will soar.

Race walking requires a great deal of effort to compete successfully. The effort comes in many forms, including a unique combination of physical exertion and mental focus. People often ask if it is hard to race walk. If time is a measure, race walking wins hands down. It is the longest footrace at the Olympics; a 50km race walk can be completed in just over 3:32 vs. running a marathon which takes just under 2:02. Therefore, race walkers must exert effort significantly longer than their running counterparts. If instead you use heart rate as a measure, race walking is pretty hard. An elite male race walker completes a 20km in under 1:20 and averages a heart rate between 180 and 190 beats per minute (bpm). For a 50km, the best in the world have an average heart rate between 160 and 170 bpm. That may seem high, but that's nothing compared to what can be achieved while working out. A young, elite race walker can clock as high as 220 bpm. Race walking gets the heart working just as well as running does, but without excessive jarring to the body. Race walking is also more difficult if you measure difficulty by calories burned. Since race walking is less efficient than running, it means race walkers burn more calories per mile than runners. Finally, if you measure difficulty by concentration, both runners and walkers push their bodies to the limit, but runners do not have to worry about being disqualified for poor form. Race walkers, on the other hand, are constantly watched, especially when they are pushing the hardest.

Given these considerations, the total exertion of race walking is arguably greater than that of running. This exertion calls for effort — a simple word with multiple meanings. To become stronger, effort is applied in the form of training; to walk faster, effort is applied in the form of exertion; to improve technique, effort is applied in the form of practice, remedial drills, concentration and, well, more practice. When we were beginning race walkers, we mistakenly thought that as we got in better shape, racing would get easier. We couldn't have been more wrong. As we trained more, our engine got bigger and the effort that we were capable of grew immensely. Remember when you just started to learn to race walk? Do you remember your legs getting really sore, but your lungs were not tired? We also remember thinking that if we just got stronger, we could cruise effortlessly along to faster times. Then one day it was as if someone flipped a switch, our legs felt better and our lungs were gasping for air. We are not alone. When you are tired and ready to succumb to the demon of fatigue, robbing you of your personal best, remember elites experience the same discomfort. Remember their effort and apply the same. As Gary Westerfield once said, "Nothing hurts more than a bad race." He was correct. The pain of exertion goes away shortly after you stop; the pain of disappointment due to a lack of effort can last a lifetime.

Still Want to Learn More?

Visit *www.racewalk.com* for a wealth of free information about race walking or to purchase our other products including the following:

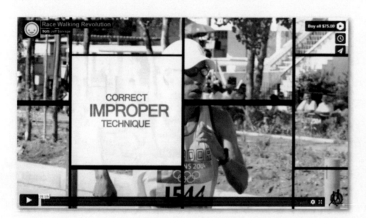

The *Race Walking Revolution* video (3 disc DVD set or streaming videos) is a comprehensive set of videos covering the basic technique of race walking, proper shoe selection, full-body strength training, extensive remedial advice and more. Over two hours and twenty minutes long, it is the most comprehensive video instruction available anywhere. It literally brings this book to life and with the exception of one of our clinics is the best way to learn how to race walk. Whether you are just learning race walking to maximize your walking workout, wishing to become a legal race walker to compete, or looking to fine tune your technique to shave minutes off your time, the *Race Walking Revolution* video is perfect to help you meet your goals. Available at *www.racewalk.com*.

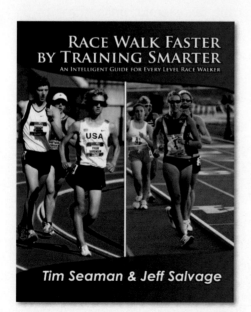

Race Walk Faster by Training Smarter is for the countless coaches who say they do not know how to coach race walking, and for every athlete interested in training for our great event. The needs of youth, high school, collegiate, elite, and masters athletes vary based on physiology and racing schedules, and one methodology cannot cover all of these intricacies. *Race Walk Faster by Training Smarter* is an entire book devoted to training. We lay out the information required for a race walker to train at any level, and we assume no prior knowledge related to endurance training. The concepts are not hard to learn. Coaches of distance runners will find many of the concepts familiar - and not surprisingly, since race walking is an endurance event within the sport of track and field. The principles behind training a race walker are not much different from the principles behind training a distance runner for races of comparable length and time. Sure, race walkers take longer to complete the same distance, but concepts like periodization, proper recovery, and peaking all apply. Available from *amazon.com*.

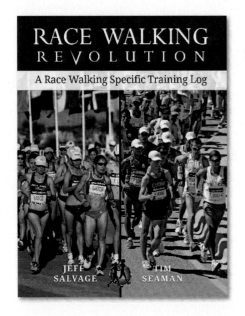

We all know we should keep a training log. It allows you to keep track of your successes and perhaps more importantly, learn from your mistakes. Some of us scribble down our workouts in an inconsistent manner, while many of us do not get beyond the new season's resolution to keep better track of our workouts. Now with **Race Walking Revolution – A Race Walking Specific Training Log**, you have a simple template-based system to record all of the pertinent details of your training and hopefully be inspired along the way.

Our training log is based on two-time Olympian Tim Seaman's personal training log. It's one that he perfected over a career that includes 47 US National titles. The log contains room for you to record workouts 7 days a week for 52 weeks of the year. There is space allowing you to record many specific aspects of your daily training as well as containing an area for more general notes each day. In addition, each week contains an area for any other notes that might not be captured within the template. Additionally, full-color photographs of elite race walkers are included every week to inspire you. At the end of the log, we include space for monthly totals, race results, and a personal records (PRs) progression. So, take a step into a champion's shoes and start your progression to a more successful walking program by filling out your training log today. Available at **www.racewalk.com**.

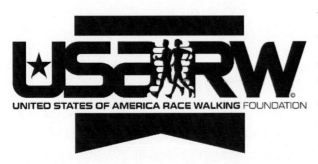

The **USA Race Walking Foundation** (USARWF), was established by Elaine P. Ward in 1992. It is a 501.c3 non-profit, tax-exempt, philanthropic organization dedicated to assisting college age and younger elite racewalkers in their quest for national and international prominence in racewalking.

USARWF's funds are generated solely through tax-deductible donations from individuals, groups, corporations, trusts, endowments, and other such entities whose common goal is to assist in the development of a strong contingent of junior and open elite athletes who are training for USA national teams, Olympic Trials, and Olympic Games.

USARWF was instrumental in funding the ARCO Olympic Training Center for racewalkers in Chula Vista, CA, in the 1990's including subsidizing the salary for the race walk coach and travel-training expenses of some of the Olympic athletes in the Sydney Games. We continued supporting athletes giving aid to virtually every Olympian since Sydney as well as financially supporting elite racewalking athletes from youth through juniors to collegiate and many post collegiate athletes.

For more information and to donate, please visit **www.usaracewalking.org**.